DOMESTIC VIOLENCE AND HEALTH

The response of the medical profession

Emma Williamson

The POLICY PRESS

First published in Great Britain in December 2000 by

The Policy Press
University of Bristol
34 Tyndall's Park Road
Bristol BS8 1PY
UK

Tel no +44 (0)117 954 6800
Fax no +44 (0)117 973 7308
E-mail tpp@bristol.ac.uk
www.policypress.org.uk

ISBN 1 86134 215 2

Emma Williamson is a Wellcome Research Fellow in the Centre for Medical
Ethics, University of Bristol.

Cover design by Qube Design Associates, Bristol.

Front cover: Photograph kindly supplied by Steve West.

Printed in Great Britain by Hobbs the Printers Ltd, Southampton.

no index,

Contents

Acknowledgements

I would like to thank a number of people for their help and support during the course of writing this book. I would like to thank my colleagues in the School for Policy Studies, at the University of Bristol. As always I would like to thank the participants of the research on which this text is based and members of the BSA Violence Against Women Study Group. I would also like to thank Professor Betsy Stanko for her extremely useful comments and suggestions. Particular thanks to Bimmy Rai, previously of DDVAG, for your professional insights and friendship. A big thank you to Stefan Bojanowski, as the saying goes "You never forget a good teacher!".

I would like to thank my friends – you know who you are – and my family, Roy, Gail, Sarah and Thomas Williamson [whose birthday I forgot while writing this book – sorry!].

A very big thank you to the editorial and production team at The Policy Press for working so hard on the original text.

And finally special thanks to Eldin Fahmy, for being there, and for restoring my faith. Thank you.

This book is dedicated to the memory of my grandmother

Hilda Williamson
1925-2000

ONE

Introduction

The purpose of this book is to investigate the medical interactions which occur between a variety of healthcare professionals and women who have experienced domestic violence. This relates specifically to the medical profession as opposed to other professionals who are accessed as part of wider help-seeking activities. Specific questions which will be addressed in this book include: whether domestic violence has undergone a process of medicalisation; whether such a process is likely to occur; what the implications of such a process are or would be; how healthcare professionals reconcile their responsibilities between the provision of healthcare and social action intended to challenge domestic violence; and finally whether women who experience domestic violence perceive the medical profession as a source of adequate help and assistance within a wider help-seeking process.

In order to address these questions, the research on which this book is based will first examine the perceptions of women who have experienced domestic violence, before focusing on the perceptions of healthcare professionals themselves. A feminist methodology was utilised in all interviews with stage one participants – women who had experienced domestic violence[1] (10 interviewees), and with second-stage participants – a range of primary healthcare practitioners (23 interviewees)[2]. The second stage participants were recruited through an earlier domestic violence and health study, the results of which are discussed in Abbott and Williamson (1999)[3]. All participants have been allocated pseudonyms.

In conjunction with examining the practical aspects of this particular medical interaction, the theoretical aim of this book is to contextualise the effects of the medical interaction in relation to the self-identity of the presenting women. These effects cannot be separated from the domestic violence itself, nor from the help seeking, in relation to other professionals, of women who experience domestic violence. As such, this book explores questions relating to the impact of medicalisation on the lives of women, and the role of professional and gender ideology on the medical interaction. It raises questions about the way in which healthcare professionals communicate, not only with one another, but with wider society, through the documentation and recording of patients' injuries and problems. Finally, this book will identify recommendations and examples of 'good practice' in order to assist the medical profession in providing an appropriate service to its female clients who have experienced domestic violence. Put very simply, this book and the research on which it is based asks, 'Do British healthcare professionals diagnose domestic violence as the primary cause of a domestic violence-related injury and how do they respond?'

Why domestic violence and health?

Although there has emerged a wide and varied domestic violence discourse since the emergence of the first women's refuge in 1972 (Dobash and Dobash, 1992), it is only very recently that research emanating from Britain has focused specifically on the role of healthcare professionals. There are several explanations as to why it has taken so long to begin to address comprehensively the issue of domestic violence and health in a British context. Following the identification of domestic violence as a serious social issue by feminists within the Women's Liberation Movement of the late 1960s and early 1970s, there emerged a 'Battered Women's Movement' whose aim was to offer crisis provision for women and children fleeing domestic violence (Dobash and Dobash, 1992). Alongside this grass-roots activism there emerged a body of research initiated by feminists to ascertain the extent, causes and responses to domestic violence, as well as other forms of violence against women (Dobash and Dobash, 1979, 1992; Bograd, 1982; Stanko, 1987; Yllo and Bograd, 1988; Herman, 1992a, 1992b; Bart and Moran, 1993; Glass, 1995). Practical or grass-roots research focused initially on the provision of refuges or safe houses for women, both for crisis and for long-term provision (Dobash and Dobash, 1992), and the initial response of the criminal justice system through the police, magistrates and judges (Radford, 1987, 1992; Stanko, 1987). A number of British researchers (Pahl, 1985, 1995; Home Office, 1989; McGibbon et al, 1989; Dobash and Dobash, 1992; Hague and Malos, 1993; McWilliams and McKiernan, 1993; Glass, 1995; Mama, 1996; Stanko et al, 1998) have identified health as an area of concern. However, this has predominantly emerged within wider research examining the help-seeking activities and support networks of women who have themselves experienced domestic violence rather than as a deliberate examination of domestic violence and health. The various reasons why domestic violence and health is now receiving specific attention include:

- The previous focus on police procedures and the response of the criminal justice system has now resulted in the adoption in some police forces of specialised domestic violence units to deal with domestic violence cases[4]. Many law enforcement and criminal justice agencies are now routinely represented within local domestic violence multi-agency initiatives, and policies and guidelines exist which are intended to improve the response of the police in particular to domestic violence[5].
- There has been a national increase of multi-agency forums to deal with domestic violence on which the representation of healthcare professionals has been poor (Hague et al, 1996). This research, in conjunction with the experiences of women's advocates, led to concerns being raised about the impact of such under-representation.
- Domestic violence as a healthcare issue has been incorporated within many international discussions of human rights issues as an area of concern to be addressed (UN, 1993a, 1993b; Lorentlen and Løkke, 1997; WHO, 1997).
- There has emerged since the 1960s an increasingly individualistic approach to the effects and causes of domestic violence which has seen an increase in therapeutic interventions, which in many cases are incorporated within existing healthcare services (Dobash and Dobash, 1992; Herman, 1992a, 1992b; Glass, 1995; Schornstein, 1997; Gondolf, 1998).
- Healthcare professions themselves are beginning to acknowledge the existence of domestic violence within their own workload, and are beginning to discuss, although predominantly within a North American context, the implications of domestic violence on their professional practice and communities generally (efor example, AMA, 1992; McAfee, 1994; Friend et al, 1998).

At present there are various individuals within Britain conducting research to ascertain the effectiveness of healthcare professionals' response to patients presenting with domestic violence-related injuries. This research includes that being conducted by healthcare professionals, professional bodies, government initiatives, domestic violence inter-agency collaborations, and feminist researchers and women's advocates. The World Health Organisation (WHO, 1997), the United Nations (UN, 1993a, 1993b), and the European Council (Lorentlen and Løkke, 1997), have all identified the importance of domestic violence for health provision on a global scale. Within Britain, following from recommendations developed at the Fourth World Conference on Women in Beijing in September 1995 (the Beijing Declaration and Platform for Action, WHO, 1997), the (previous) British Conservative government introduced recommendations for the implementation of national multi-agency professional forums to deal more adequately with the issue of domestic violence (Home Office, 1995). This inter-agency circular included the medical and health professions, as the following quotation illustrates:

> In order to promote an effective health care response to the incidence of domestic violence and child abuse, it is good practice for purchasers and provider units to consider taking into account the needs of domestic violence victims when planning the purchase and delivery of services. (Home Office, 1995, p 22)

Despite this international and national governmental impetus encouraging healthcare professionals to address the issue of domestic violence, research conducted to evaluate the effectiveness of the government's inter-agency initiatives found that the representation of healthcare professionals on such inter-agency forums was "at best poor" (Hague et al, 1996). Considering that this particular research was examining the response of a diverse range of professionals to domestic violence, it is pertinent to question whether there are specific reasons for the poor representation of health professions within such inter-agency initiatives.

Over the last two years the British government has begun to address this issue by incorporating health within domestic violence crime reduction initiatives (Davidson et al, 2000). These policy initiatives are an important move forward within Britain and have culminated in the publication of a Department of Health resource manual specifically targeting health practitioners, which was published in March 2000[6] (DoH, 2000). This manual brings together guidelines developed by a number of health organisations, including: the British Medical Association (BMA, 1998), the Royal College of Obstetrics and Gynaecology (Friend et al, 1998), the Royal College of General Practice (Heath, 1992) and the British Association of Accident and Emergency Medicine (BAAMA, 1994). The Department of Health's resource manual is particularly useful as it sets out guidance for practitioners in relation to specific issues relevant to the interaction which occurs between women who have experienced domestic violence and healthcare professionals. In particular, it addresses facts about domestic violence, information pertaining to the recognition, screening and treatment of domestic violence, the role of inter-agency fora, and training. While this manual is a positive move forward in that it makes recommendations for policy and practice development, it is still unclear how such information will impact on a profession which has so far, within Britain in particular, avoided calls for greater understanding of the issue of domestic violence. The research on which this book is based was conducted prior to the publication of this manual, and as such is a valuable source of baseline data with which to monitor changes which may occur as a result of its dissemination.

The most important reason why researchers are beginning to address the issue of domestic violence and health is that women who experience domestic violence use health services as part of a wider help-seeking process (Stark and Flitcraft, 1996; Stanko et al, 1998). The importance of healthcare professionals within the wider help-seeking processes of women experiencing domestic violence was acknowledged in Britain as early as the mid-1980s (Pahl, 1985, 1995; Home Office, 1989; McGibbon et al, 1989; Dobash and Dobash, 1992; Hague and Malos, 1993; McWilliams and McKiernan, 1993; Glass, 1995; Mama, 1996; Stanko et al, 1998). This makes the lack of substantial research on this issue, until very recently, particularly interesting. Although British healthcare professionals have been criticised for not being adequately represented within inter-agency forums, a number are beginning to address this issue (Llewellyn et al, 1995; Richardson and Feder, 1996; Friend et al, 1998), albeit several years later than their North American colleagues.

All of these factors have culminated in an increase in research focusing on domestic violence and health within Britain. Due to the manner in which it has emerged, this body of research is often associated with local domestic violence inter-agency initiatives and therefore has local as well as national and international ramifications[7].

International research

While the emergence of the above research is extremely interesting and commendable, it comes 18 years after the emergence of a substantial body of research emanating from North America (Bograd, 1982; Stark and Flitcraft, 1982, 1995, 1996; Goldberg and Tomlanovich, 1984; Klingbeil and Boyd, 1984; Kurz, 1987; Kurz and Stark, 1988; Randall, 1990a, 1990b; Cascardi et al, 1992; Koss, 1994; Kornblit, 1994; Abbott et al, 1995; Delahunta, 1995; Johnson, 1995; Finkler, 1997; Fishbach and Herbert, 1997; Desjarlais and Kleinman, 1997; Schornstein, 1997; Gondolf, 1998). Although not as prolific as the literature from North

America, international research also exists focusing specifically on domestic violence and health (Heise, 1994; Olavarrieta and Soleto, 1996). The North American literature regarding domestic violence and the response of the medical profession includes articles by various professional health providers including the nursing professions (Campbell, 1992; Varvaro and Lasko, 1993; Butler, 1995; Denham, 1995; Fishwick, 1995), dentists (McDowell, 1994), prenatal care professionals (Webster et al, 1994), army medical providers (Hamlin et al, 1991), paediatric service providers (Wolfe and Korsch, 1994; Zuckerman et al, 1995) as well as community pharmacists (Taylor, 1994). All these professionals urge their colleagues to deal adequately with the issue of domestic violence in an attempt to reinforce the legal position that domestic violence is a crime and unacceptable, as well as offering the appropriate help and support to those on the receiving end. It is within the context of this research that this book, and the research on which it is based, is located.

Definitions

In order to focus the research on which this book is based, domestic violence throughout will refer to the *physical, emotional, psychological and sexual abuse of women by their intimate male partners and ex-partners whether married or living as a couple.* This definition is intended to define the concept of domestic violence sufficiently for it to be meaningful without excluding the meanings women themselves may attribute to the experience.

This working definition is gender specific, in that it refers to women who experience domestic violence which is perpetrated by male partners. This is deliberate as it is predominantly women who are the 'victims' of domestic violence. The statistical prevalence of domestic violence on women will be examined in detail shortly; however, quantitative data illustrates that, of the 4,764 incidents of domestic violence responded to by the Police Domestic Violence Unit of Derbyshire Constabulary's D division in 1997, 4,366 (91.6%) involved incidents where the 'victim' was female[8] (Derbyshire Constabulary, 'D' division, 1997). These official statistics demonstrate that women are significantly more likely to be the 'victim' of a serious offence between spouses than men.

Taking a gender–specific definition of domestic violence within this book is not intended to undermine the individual experiences of men who experience domestic violence perpetrated by their female partners, nor the occurrence of violence within homosexual relationships. The author recognises that patriarchal power is mediated and experienced through a number of forms of oppression. However, if healthcare professionals are unable to treat adequately women who present with domestic violence-related injuries, and who by far account for the largest group affected by domestic violence, then it is unlikely that healthcare professionals will be adequately informed to deal with 'others' who experience such violence and who may be subject to very different social stereotypes and cultural myths associated with being placed in that position. Any references within this book to intimate relationships will therefore refer to heterosexual relationships unless otherwise stated[9].

As mentioned at the outset, this research does not utilise the terms 'victim' or 'survivor', as they are problematic in relation to the cultural meanings attached to each. Such a distinction also perpetuates the dichotomy of identity categories available to women who experience violence, which is not helpful. This is particularly pertinent when considering health, as the terms 'victim' and 'survivor' are often utilised within the therapeutic interventions this book seeks to examine.

Finally, this book is concerned with the response of a range of healthcare professionals to domestic violence. There are very clear differentiations which are relevant, however, in relation to specific health practitioners. The concept of a gendered medical hierarchy is addressed within this text and distinctions are made between the responses of specific healthcare providers. Nevertheless, despite these differences, when considered within a wider inter-agency professional context these health practitioners share a number of ideological perspectives which do differentiate them from others working with this issue[10].

Chapters

As this first chapter has argued, there is a need for British research which examines the issue of domestic violence and health, and which contextualises such research within the vast body of feminist-based domestic violence research. This chapter has identified a number of reasons why domestic violence and health has not been addressed until recently within a British context and has defined the specific terms of reference which will be utilised throughout this text, bearing in mind the often complex and problematic implications of such terms. This book is intended for use by a range of health professionals, particularly in relation to the experiences of the individual female research participants. These experiential accounts, however, must be located within the research identified above. Only through viewing women's individual experiences within a wider framework of national and international policy and professional practice can we collectively challenge abuses of power which have serious social repercussions for societies around the world.

Chapter Two examines the literature introduced above. It considers: the statistical prevalence of domestic violence-related injuries; dilemmas in screening, policy and protocols; feminist criticisms of the health interaction; stigmatisation; cultural myths; psychiatric labelling; secondary versus primary diagnosis of violence; and issues relating therapy and disease categorisations. This chapter focuses specifically on domestic violence and health, but begins to consider the themes of medicalisation and professionalism which are prevalent throughout this text.

The results of the research on which this book is based have been separated into three distinct sections. The first of these contains interview extracts from the stage one participants, women who have themselves experienced domestic violence. Part One contains three chapters. Chapter Three examines the types of injuries which the participating women sustained as a result of domestic violence and contextualises this data with information from other research. Chapter Four looks in depth at the perceptions of the stage one participants in relation to their treatment experiences. These treatment experiences include: giving information and advice; counselling; prescription drugs; self-medication; documentation; and issues relating to the perceptions of the participating women. These perceptions are demonstrated through generic and specific examples of bad practice which included a lack of validation of experiences, blaming women, and a lack of advocacy. Chapter Five looks at the wider help-seeking activities of the participating women. This chapter focuses on the police, social services, teachers, and the criminal justice system. The importance of inter-agency fora is stressed throughout this text, as it is crucial that healthcare professionals understand that women access them for assistance as part of wider help-seeking strategies which involve other professionals. Each section has a summary, which highlights in bullet form the key areas for consideration. Part One is important, as it is essential that practitioners and policy makers consider how their efforts are perceived by those they are intended to help.

Part Two of this text focuses on the perceptions of healthcare professionals. Chapters Six and Seven begin by contextualising the health interaction in relation to practitioners' knowledge of domestic violence. This knowledge is presented in relation to definitions of clinicians' roles, both generally and specifically to domestic violence, definitions of domestic violence, and explanations of domestic violence.

abuse to look for the psychological
pressures psy.
mental health -

Chapter Seven also examines how healthcare professionals perceive patients who present with domestic violence-related injuries. While some of these perceptions come from clinical experience, they demonstrate how practitioners consider domestic violence beyond the individual medical (health) encounter. Chapters Eight, Nine and Ten are concerned with the clinical experiences of the participating healthcare professionals in relation to their interactions with women who present with domestic violence-related injuries. These chapters consider: the identification of physical injuries; the differentiation between physical and non-physical injuries; treatment options as preferred and utilised by the participating healthcare professionals; and issues of the documentation and naming of domestic violence. Throughout Part Two the perceptions of the participating healthcare professionals are compared with the experiences of women illustrated in Part One.

Part Three brings together key issues raised by both groups of participants to examine relationships between the different health professions, participation within wider inter-agency initiatives, and training. While recommendations are made throughout the text, Part Three in particular is intended to offer practical suggestions for the improvement of medical services offered to women experiencing violence. A range of practical tools is examined in Chapter Thirteen, which can be utilised in both training and clinical practice.

Finally, Chapter Fourteen will re-examine the key findings of the research on which this book is based. It revisits theoretical discussions which emerge in all three parts, and reiterates the key recommendations which appear at the end of each section. This chapter is also followed by useful information which can be accessed by health professionals, students and teachers to improve their knowledge of domestic violence and health, thereby giving women who experience domestic violence an appropriate and improved service.

Notes

[1] Due to the problematic nature of naming both domestic violence and those who experience it, the terms 'victim' and 'survivor' are not routinely used in this book. As an alternative, women who experience domestic violence are named as such.

[2] For a discussion of the methodological issues relevant to this research see Williamson (2000).

[3] For a detailed list of the research participants, see Appendix 1, Tables A1 and A2.

[4] These units come under different names; for example, within the London Borough of Hammersmith and Fulham there exists a Vulnerable Persons Unit (Domestic Violence Forum: Hammersmith and Fulham, 1998).

[5] Bridgeman and Hobbs (1997), Plotnikoff and Woolfson (1998), Hanmer et al (1999), Kelly et al (1999).

[6] See Appendix 2: Useful information and contacts, for details of how to obtain this manual.

[7] For example, this particular study has been conducted with the support of Derby Domestic Violence Action Group.

[8] These statistics include all types of familial violence responded to by the Police Domestic Violence Unit.

[9] For a discussion of the specific issues relating to domestic violence within lesbian and gay/bisexual relationships see Coleman (1994) and Letellier (1994) respectively.

[10] For a list of the healthcare professionals represented in stage two, see Appendix 1, Table A2.

TWO

Domestic violence and the medical profession

Much of the British domestic violence and health research emanates from localised studies focusing on women's wider experiences of domestic violence (Pahl, 1985, 1995; Home Office, 1989; McGibbon et al, 1989; Dobash and Dobash, 1992; Hague and Malos, 1993; McWilliams and McKiernan, 1993; Glass, 1995; Mama, 1996; Stanko et al, 1998). Alternatively, research has emerged from health practitioners in North America (Bograd, 1982; Stark and Flitcraft, 1982, 1995, 1996; Goldberg and Tomlanovich, 1984; Klingbeil and Boyd, 1984; Kurz, 1987; Kurz and Stark, 1988; Randall, 1990a, 1990b; Cascardi et al, 1992; Kornblit, 1994; Koss, 1994; Abbott et al, 1995; Delahunta, 1995; Johnson, 1995; Finkler, 1997; Fishbach and Herbert, 1997; Desjarlais and Kleinman, 1997; Schornstein, 1997; Gondolf, 1998). As such, much of the specific research focusing on domestic violence and health has emerged from feminist concerns rather than from purely medical considerations of domestic violence as a health issue. The research on which this book is based is intended to contribute to, and build upon, the following body of knowledge and will address a number of the key issues which such research has identified as central to a consideration of domestic violence and health.

Statistical relevance, injuries and prevalence

Although the occurrence of domestic violence is statistically high, there are few needs assessment studies which identify domestic violence as a specific health issue, particularly in Britain. The reasons for this lack of knowledge have been outlined already and include the previous focus on responses from other statutory and voluntary agencies. Focusing on the response of the medical profession to domestic violence is important, as many women will require healthcare services, whether they utilise them or not, for a diverse range of injuries (both physical and non-physical) which are caused by domestic violence. Various healthcare professionals and researchers, again predominantly from North America, have identified the diverse range of symptoms which they believe are related to domestic violence.

Box 1: Domestic violence-related injuries

Abrasions, lacerations, contusions, fractures, sprains, strains, alterations in nutrition, sleep disturbances, drug overdoses, suicide attempts, substance abuse, miscarriage, early labour, anxiety, depression (Johnson, 1979; Bergman and Brismar, 1991; Denham, 1995; Stark and Flitcraft, 1995), facial injuries, particularly to the lips, eyes and teeth, hair loss and perforated tympanic membrane (Dym, 1995), post traumatic stress disorder (Herman, 1992a, 1992b; Saunders, 1994; Stark and Flitcraft, 1995), abdominal or pelvic pain, headaches, gastrointestinal disorders, low birth rate (Parsons et al, 1995), haematoma, fractures, inflammation, penetrating puncture wounds and haemorrhages (Easteal and Easteal, 1992; Bates et al, 1995; Stanko et al, 1998).

Box 1 identifies the types of injuries women who experience domestic violence have inflicted upon them by male partners and which they present to healthcare professionals. One of the aims of the research on which this text is based is to examine how health professionals deal with the issue of domestic violence when it is clear that there is such diversity in the types of domestic violence-related injuries they may be presented with.

In terms of the statistical relevance of women presenting with domestic violence-related injuries, the studies which do exist demonstrate that domestic violence is a serious social problem which has significant healthcare implications. The first extract below is from North America, the second from a recent British study.

> Whereas physicians saw 1 in 35 of their patients as battered, a more accurate approximation is 1 in 4. (Stark and Flitcraft, 1995, p 10)

> In total, 60 percent of the women said that they had experienced some sort of abuse. In all, one in nine (eleven percent) reported violence which is serious enough to require medical attention in the past year. (Stanko et al, 1998, p 21)

These statistics highlight the extent of the problem of domestic violence. Both quotations demonstrate that domestic violence is a serious health issue which needs to be examined further, particularly within a British context. To reiterate, the World Health Organisation stated in 1997 that "Violence against women is a public health problem. It can be prevented" (WHO, 1997). This assertion can also be found in other international policy statements which address the issue of domestic violence and health:

...former Surgeon General C. Everett Koop declared violence against women as the number one health problem of American women in 1985. (Cascardi et al, 1992, p 1178)

Healthy People 2000 identified violent and abusive behaviour as a national health concern and a priority area for intervention. (Denham, 1995, p 13)

Whether the medical profession is suited to dealing with domestic violence-related injuries or not, the fact that so many women present with such injuries (Pahl, 1985, 1995; Home Office, 1989; McGibbon et al, 1989; Hague and Malos, 1993; McWilliams and McKiernan, 1993; Stanko et al, 1998) is problematic both for the healthcare worker, the presenting women and for the medical profession itself. The list of injuries, included above, which have been identified by health professionals as relating to domestic violence includes both physical and non-physical injuries. This differentiation is important as it demonstrates that healthcare professionals are aware that they are likely to be presented with injuries which go beyond those that can be seen, such as bruises, fractures and cuts.

In addition to physical injuries, abused women frequently experience anxiety, fatigue, dependency, depression, sleeping and eating disorders, chronic pain, and other problems that result from living with constant stress. (Butler, 1995, p 55)

How healthcare professionals deal with a woman presenting domestic violence-related injuries and how they perceive and treat non-physical injuries caused by domestic violence will be discussed in Chapter Eight. However, this literature is vital in clearly identifying that the physical and non-physical injuries which women sustain as a result of domestic violence are diverse, with a wide range of health implications to be taken into consideration. While acknowledging this diversity is important, it has also been possible to identify those injuries which are most frequently presented to the medical profession and which have domestic violence as their primary cause.

The most common injuries were bruising, fractures and cuts. The parts of the body most frequently injured were the face, head and arms. Eighteen per cent of women reported experiencing a fracture

> in the most recent episode and 55 per cent of women experienced a
> haematoma. (Bates et al, 1995, p 297)

Such research, while identifying the more common injuries sustained
through domestic violence, could become problematic if it hierarchises
the seriousness of an injury in relation to its location in a biomedical
framework, rather than within a framework defined by the presenting
woman herself. For example, while bruises, fractures, and cuts may be
easily identified, depression and anxiety may be considered more
damaging to overall well-being from the woman's own perspective. Such
an identification of the most common injuries may also obscure the
need for healthcare professionals to consider the cause of injuries within
their female adult caseloads on a generic basis. While some research has
examined the prevalence of presentation of domestic violence-related
injuries in specific medical settings (Stark and Flitcraft, 1982, 1996;
Goldberg and Tomlanovich, 1984; Kurz, 1987; Kurz and Stark, 1988),
this literature has generally failed to identify significant demographic
factors identifying which women who experience domestic violence
are more likely to present related injuries. This is important, since it is
widely acknowledged (Dobash and Dobash, 1992) that domestic violence
crosses boundaries of race, nationality and economic status.

The only demographic variation which also identifies a specific
medical setting where violence-related injuries are more likely to be
presented is within pregnancy:

> Pregnancy is a high-risk period during which violence may begin
> or escalate, harming the fetus as well as the mother. Approximately
> 23% of obstetrical patients are in abusive relationships. (Stark and
> Flitcraft, 1996, p 203)

While this research and that of others (Webster et al, 1994; Chez, 1994;
Denham, 1994; Norton et al, 1995; Schornstein, 1997) identifies that
women are more likely to experience abuse during pregnancy, either as
a first incident of abusive behaviour or the escalation of violence already
present within the relationship, health professionals still appear reluctant
to address the issue. Focusing on the interaction by health professionals
within this statistically relevant medical setting, professionals have offered
numerous reasons why they have not recognised and intervened in cases
of abuse and violence. These include:

(1) close identification with patients (39%), especially by female physicians with a history of abuse or by a physician with socioeconomic status similar to that of patients; (2) fear of offending patients (55%); (3) feelings of inadequacy and frustration in providing appropriate interventions (50%) and lack of training (55%); (4) inability of physician to control the situation and "cure" the problem (42%); and (5) lack of time to deal appropriately with abuse (71%). (Parsons et al, 1995, p 385)

All these issues will be discussed in relation to the research on which this book is based. However, the above research demonstrates the problems which are faced by the medical profession, as they find it difficult to address the occurrence of violence within medical settings identified by their own research. This raises questions about how seriously healthcare professionals take the issue of domestic violence. It also questions why healthcare professionals are conducting such research if they are reluctant to put the findings into practice.

Screening, policies and protocols

Those professionals who have identified domestic violence as a serious problem in their everyday practice (Hadley, 1992; Chez, 1994; McAfee, 1994; Dym, 1995; Denham, 1995; Llewellyn et al, 1995; Parsons et al, 1995) have been concerned that a uniform medical approach to the problem does not exist and that domestic violence is often missed because practitioners are uncomfortable dealing with patients presenting with domestic violence injuries. Some practitioners, however (Doner, 1994; Denham, 1995; Dym, 1995; Fishwick, 1995), have been reflexive in their consideration of the impact of domestic violence on both their personal and professional practice. They have outlined the feelings which dealing with domestic violence elicits. They define the personal issues a practitioner will need to address, in order to ensure that the services they offer women presenting with violence-related injuries are based on giving the best possible care. They also identify that practitioners may avoid the issue because it is difficult, time consuming, inconvenient or uncomfortable:

> Nurses have a responsibility to respond proactively to this national problem based upon their citizenry and professional accountability. (Denham, 1995, p 19)

The reasons why some practitioners are addressing the issue of domestic violence are admirable. Where there has been recognition of the personal, social and professional implications of domestic violence as a serious health issue, the discussions which have emerged have been extremely productive. With the increase, in Britain, of guidelines for specific medical professions (Heath, 1992; BAAMA, 1994; BMA, 1998; Friend et al, 1998; DoH, 2000), it is relevant to question whether such guidelines can be implemented without basic awareness training which addresses the wider role of practitioners in patient interactions and in wider society. Just as domestic violence exists within a social discourse which encompasses political and social power and control, so too does the medical interaction exist within a medical discourse which is subject to the same power dynamics. The medical discourse has also emerged within an historical framework where its existence has implicated women in specific gendered roles (Cloward and Piven, 1979; Stark, 1982; Riessman, 1983; Oakley, 1993).

In relation to the development of guidelines and policies, healthcare professionals have also examined issues relating to screening women for domestic violence (Tilden and Shepherd, 1987; Lazzaro and McFarlane, 1991; AMA, 1992; Hendricks-Matthews, 1993; Sheridan, 1993; Butler, 1995; Delahunta, 1995; DoH, 2000).

> Routine screening for partner abuse directed toward all women is a reasonable expectation based on the widespread occurrence of domestic violence. (Butler, 1995, p 57)

While those practitioners who acknowledge the widespread occurrence of domestic violence often advocate health screening for domestic violence, particularly within prenatal healthcare (Webster et al, 1994; Chez, 1994; Parsons et al, 1995), there is a sense of unease in much of this literature which is based on the reluctance of healthcare professionals to screen their patients for a social problem, even though this social problem has widespread health implications. This is evident in the suggestion within the Department of Health's recently published resource manual (DoH, 2000) that selective screening may be an appropriate step forward. The above literature clarifies the responsibility of healthcare professionals to: deal effectively with domestic violence and health; examine general principles of intervention (Goodwin, 1985; AMA, 1992; Hadley, 1992; Straus and Smith, 1993); implement domestic violence protocols/policies (Langford, 1990; AMA, 1992; Hoag-Apel, 1994); and finally, address training (AMA, 1992; Schoonmaker and Shull, 1994) which is intended to ensure the adequate provision of services for women experiencing domestic violence. As with policy development, screening for domestic violence has inherent within it a range of contradictions which fit uneasily within medical discourse. These contradictions relate to the concept of 'health absolutism' (found within holistic/person-led models of healthcare) (Gallagher and Ferrante, 1987) and its impact on the medicalisation of social problems and the professionalisation of medicine itself (Davis, 1979; Stark, 1982; Turner, 1995). For a more detailed analysis of the impact of these concepts on the medical profession, see Williamson (1999).

Feminist criticisms of the health interaction

As suggested earlier, one of the reasons why domestic violence and health are receiving attention from researchers in Britain at this time is the fact that women are utilising such services (Pahl, 1985; McGibbon et al, 1989; McWilliams and McKiernan, 1993). As such, domestic violence advocates have been central in engaging healthcare professionals within debates about their current service provision[1]. From the concerns which advocates have expressed, many North American feminist researchers have challenged the medical profession's response to 'victims' of domestic violence. This research has identified problems, some of which relate specifically to the treatment of domestic violence-related injuries, and others which relate to the generic complaint that women's 'problems' are medicalised and marginalised within medical discourse and practice (Stark, 1982; Riessman, 1983; Oakley, 1984). The following sections address specific issues relating to feminist concerns and identify research which has examined the medical response to domestic violence.

Stigmatisation

Kurz (1987) conducted research focusing on domestic violence and the medical profession which, through participant observation, examined the responses of medical staff to women who presented themselves with domestic violence-related injuries. The results of this study demonstrated that only 11% of women presenting themselves with injuries relating to domestic violence received an 'adequate response', 49% received a partial response, and 40% no response at all in relation to the issue of domestic violence and the associated injuries they were presenting to medical staff. While these statistics are interesting in themselves, the reasons medical staff gave for responding in specific cases are perhaps more informative. The reasons and justifications given by members of staff when questioned about incidents which resulted in partial or no response were that the women being treated by staff were perceived to be 'evasive', 'purposely vague' and 'inconsistent'. These 'traits' resulted in medical staff identifying these women as having 'stigmatising qualities' which enabled staff to focus on the personality of the woman rather than the problems and effects of domestic violence.

This process of stigmatising the presenting women can be seen in relation to the ways in which society generally individualises the problem of domestic violence. Individualising domestic violence in conjunction with concepts of gender and race may also explain how racism and sexism are acted out within systems which enable individualisation to occur, while seemingly advocating equality for all within generalised protocols. Some staff in Kurz's study (1987) also commented that they considered domestic violence to be a personal problem in which they had no right to intervene. This is strikingly similar to the response of other professional groups who have been studied, for example the police, who also explained their lack of action by making a distinction between the public and private spheres (Radford, 1987; Stanko, 1988). Within the medical profession, however, the social control function of the 'sick role' enables healthcare professionals to identify 'good' and 'bad' patients, some of whom are worthy of treatment, and others who are stigmatised (Jeffery, 1979). This occurs for a number of reasons, one being that professionals often compare the behaviour of patients in relation to their own experiences as individuals:

> Observers who have never experienced prolonged terror and who have no understanding of coercive methods of control presume that they would show greater courage and resistance than the victim in similar circumstances. Hence the common tendency to account for the victim's behaviour by seeking flaws in her personality or moral character. (Herman, 1992a, p 115)

It is for this reason that an acknowledgement of the personal, professional and social responsibility to deal with domestic violence is important.

Cultural myths

Bograd (1982), starting from an ideologically feminist position, took the perspective that women who have experienced domestic violence continue to use health settings, despite the fact that clinical intervention is based on male-defined cultural myths about women generally and women who have experienced domestic violence in particular. Bograd identified four major myths on which such medical interventions are based. These myths were that (a) battering is rare, (b) that women are battered due to psychopathological factors either of the batterer or the battered, (c) that women are responsible for men's behaviour (for example as the guardians of men's morality), and (d) that violence is an expectable (if not acceptable) part of the experience of being a woman (Bograd, 1982). Bograd suggests that these myths influence the way in which medical staff react to women who present themselves with violence-related injuries. Indeed, they can clearly be seen as a valid explanation of why the healthcare professionals within Kurz's study were able to define some women as worthy of an adequate response and others as unworthy, through a stigmatising process. The myths Bograd identifies include: myths specifically about domestic violence, gender-differentiated socialisation and expected gender roles – myths which perpetuate the concept that individualising, and thus depoliticising, the issue of domestic violence is acceptable.

The synthesis of stigmatisation with gendered cultural myths in domestic violence cases clearly relates to the concept of the sick role. This concept is most frequently associated with the work of Talcott Parsons (1951) and relates to the way in which individuals manage ill health in relation to wider social structures and responsibilities within societies. The sick role encompasses a number of components. First, the sick role legitimates abdication of social responsibility for the duration of the illness. Second, the abdication of social and familial responsibilities is dependent on the seeking of professional help and advice. Third, the individual is responsible for assisting in the recovery process, through adherence to the professional recommendations they receive. Finally, there is an expectation that individuals seek help from specifically trained, and therefore legitimated, health providers (Turner, 1995). As such, the sick role relates to both the social control function of the medical discourse and the individual relationship between the health provider and patient. In relation to domestic violence and health, the appropriation of the sick role is the mechanism by which social control functions. This has implications for the type of medical response which patients receive, in terms of the level of patient responsibility assumed by the practitioner (for a more detailed discussion of the sick role in relation to domestic violence, see Williamson, 1999). Building on the theories of Parsons, Jeffery (1979) examined the moral evaluations which take place within the appropriation of the sick role in relation to interactions between medical staff and patients. Jeffery was particularly interested in the way health professionals use moral evaluations to label certain types of patients as 'rubbish' (for example, tramps, suicide attempts and so on). Such patients, Jeffery suggests, do not fit adequately within the sick role and thus are not treated or are treated badly. This sets up a binary opposition in which legitimate and illegitimate health states are opposed to one another, one being more desirable and positive than the other. Jeffery is suggesting that it is only those who do not legitimately fit within the role of the legitimate sick patient whose illness and behaviour is considered deviant through the stigmatisation of their behaviour as inappropriate (Goffman, 1968; Becker and McCall, 1990). Again, this has very clear implications for women presenting to medical practitioners with domestic violence-related injuries, particularly if the medical discourse within which the interaction takes place has inherent within it gendered cultural stereotypes.

Within the above studies both Kurz (1987) and Bograd (1982) demonstrate how gendered ideology and concepts of cultural deviancy permeate the medical discourse and subsequently the possibilities of the appropriation of the sick role. From this literature we can begin to observe how women who experience domestic violence are located within the medical discourse through the mechanisms of social control which function within it.

Quasi-psychiatric labels

Quite startling results were obtained in an empirical study conducted by Kurz and Stark (1988), when they examined medical records in both New Haven and Philadelphia in the US. They found that domestic violence was significantly under-reported, and, more alarmingly, 80% of women who did inform the clinician that their injuries were the result of domestic violence were not referred to a special team which the hospital itself had formed to address this problem. In relation to medical records, Kurz and Stark (1988) also found that women who identified themselves as having experienced domestic violence were more likely to have 'quasi-pyschiatric' labels attributed to them.

> Staff respond to women they see as 'true victims'. The women have to be polite, have no discrediting attributes, and, in addition, staff members have to feel that some unfortunate event has happened to them. (Kurz, 1987, p 73)

Concerns over the misdiagnosis of psychological symptoms demonstrated by women who have experienced domestic violence (Dutton and Painter, 1981; Walker, 1989, 1991; Herman, 1992a, 1992b; Saunders, 1994; Gondolf, 1998) have led to the advocated use of the post-traumatic stress disorder (PTSD) schedule in domestic violence cases. These researchers believe that advocating the use of the PTSD schedule will help to ensure that psychiatric symptoms are considered in relation to victimisation rather than as isolated psychiatric symptoms. Studies have found that PTSD, as measured by standardised instruments, is present in approximately 45-55% of small samples of women who have experienced domestic violence and who subsequently access battered women's programs (Housekamp and Foy, 1991). This figure rises to over 75% in open-ended clinical evaluations of women who are in immediate crisis (Astin et al, 1993). The PTSD schedule identifies a number of symptoms which are frequently misdiagnosed in domestic violence cases. These include avoidance symptoms (for example, amnesia, dissociative episodes, withdrawal and depression) and intrusive symptoms (for example, explosive anger, flashbacks, anxiety and hyperactivity) (Gondolf, 1998). In relation to misdiagnosis, it has been suggested that:

> These extremes [avoidance and intrusive symptoms] taken separately suggest major disorders. These extremes taken together suggest a person with PTSD coping with an unpredictable and threatening environment. (Gondolf, 1998, p 86)

While the theoretical advocacy of the PTSD (as a disease categorisation) is intended to prevent the misdiagnosis of women's psychological symptoms, in practice identifying psychological symptoms in relation to domestic violence is often problematic for mental healthcare professionals (Gondolf, 1998). If a patient is considered in relation to cultural myths and stereotypes (identified above), which minimise her experiences of violence and abuse, then it is possible for healthcare professionals to diagnose a woman's psychological symptoms in relation to psychiatric problems which subsequently minimise the role and impact of domestic violence. The ways in which cultural myths impact on the diagnostic process result in a secondary rather than primary diagnosis of domestic violence.

Secondary versus primary diagnosis

Several researchers (Bograd, 1982; Stark and Flitcraft, 1982; Klingbeil and Boyd, 1984; Klingbeil, 1986) have examined the way in which domestic violence is frequently ignored as the primary diagnosis of domestic violence-related injuries. The result of false diagnosis is, according to Klingbeil and Boyd (1984), that women are being prescribed minor tranquillisers without explanation. The 'illness' or 'displayed traits' for which the medication is prescribed then becomes significant and the issue of domestic violence is relegated yet further in relation to the injury and the woman's individual personality.

> Although few doctors agreed with the prescription of tranquillisers to spouse assault victims, it is noteworthy that tranquillisers were prescribed by 83% of ACT [Australian Capital Territory] general practitioners consulted by a sample of victims. (Easteal and Easteal, 1992, p 225)

Already we can observe similarities in the treatment of women who experience domestic violence and the treatment of women generally within medical interactions. The medicalisation of women's biological functions has resulted in the medicalisation of many aspects of women's everyday lives:

> The medicalisation of unhappiness as depression is one of the great disasters of the twentieth century, and it is a disaster that has had, and still has, a very big impact on women. (Oakley, 1993, p 8)

Focusing specifically on medical interactions which concern the psychiatric and psychological diagnosis of women, theorists (Riessman, 1983; Miles, 1991; Herman, 1992a; Oakley, 1993) have found that women are more likely to be diagnosed as experiencing psychiatric problems than men, even when they present with essentially the same symptoms (Oakley, 1993). While this appears a very serious health issue, the same researchers found that these psychiatric 'problems' are more likely to be treated by the doctor, rather than a specifically trained psychiatrist, and when referred to a psychiatrist are more likely to be seen on an out-patient basis (NIMH, 1981; Miles, 1988, 1991). Clearly, therefore, the medicalisation of women's illnesses as psychological in origin derives from the diagnoses which women are more likely to receive. It is suggested that this tendency to psychologise women is a result of the medicalisation of women as more 'natural' (bearing in mind the binary oppositions found within the Cartesian duality), and therefore biologically driven (Riessman, 1983). This in itself is evident within the medicalisation of menstruation and pregnancy, 'normal' everyday biological functions which constitute the basis of many interactions between women and healthcare professionals. The alternative reason why women are diagnosed as suffering from illnesses which require psychiatric diagnosis is that they do actually have more psychologically-based illnesses. Theorists who have considered this perspective (Miles, 1991; Oakley, 1993) suggest that it is women's oppression within patriarchal society which accounts for women's greater stress and, thus, psychiatric illness. It is evident also that women's illness is labelled psychological even when a woman presents with the same symptoms as a male patient whose illness is not psychologised (Miles, 1991). The tendency to individualise and attribute psychiatric labels to diagnose women's symptoms is evident in the domestic violence studies above (Stark and Flitcraft, 1982).

The major issues which emerge from an examination of the North American empirical and theoretical research into this field are that women are perceived in relation to the individual qualities medical staff perceive them to have or not to have. There is a serious problem with domestic violence being relegated to a position of secondary diagnosis rather than being perceived as the cause of injury requiring a primary diagnosis in its own right. Also highlighted is the issue of medical staff not referring women who have experienced domestic violence to special hospital teams set up to deal with this issue. This last point questions the effectiveness of protocols intended to improve services to women experiencing domestic violence. This final body of research raises the most crucial question which needs to be addressed within the research on which this book is based, which is, 'Do British healthcare professionals diagnose domestic violence as the primary cause of injury?'

Therapy and disease categorisations

It is possible that the problems identified in the previous sections exist because the issue of domestic violence as a health concern cannot be easily fitted within a biomedical concept of health due to the social and gendered origins of domestic violence. Concepts such as 'the battered spouse syndrome' have now been included within disease categorisations of illness through an extended concept of PTSD (Herman, 1992a, 1992b). It is necessary, therefore, to examine whether this represents a move towards the medicalisation of domestic violence. Furthermore, it is pertinent to question whether this will result in the provision of better services for women who have experienced domestic violence, or whether such a discourse will result in individual women being stigmatised due to the reliance on biological explanations for women's well-being.

Stark and Flitcraft (1982) use the term of a 'battering syndrome cycle' to identify the processes which a woman who has experienced domestic violence enters on presenting such injuries to the medical profession. While they use this concept to describe the effects it has on women who have experienced domestic violence, they do not adequately challenge the implications of advocating such a theory. As has already been discussed in Chapter One, the concept of describing women who experience domestic violence as 'victims' is extremely problematic, as is the related concept of 'survivor'. It becomes even more problematic when looking at the medical profession, since issues of mental health are often invoked as a result of women being stigmatised in terms of their personality. Such a focus, which has been identified as grounded in wider social concepts of gender ideology, results in women's behaviour being considered problematic within a medical and mental health framework.

Herman (1992a, 1992b), while investigating the processes and experiences of 'victimage', focuses specifically on domestic violence. She challenges the idea that there are any differences in the traumatic effects experienced by individuals within the public or private sphere. She suggests that experiences of trauma within both spheres are based on the same psychological processes, which affect notions of 'selfhood' and therefore well-being. She is challenging, therefore, the concept that women who experience domestic violence should be judged or their behaviour considered inappropriate. Herman also challenges the notion of 'learned helplessness', which a 'battering syndrome cycle' implies, as she suggests that the 'victim' is more alert, and the processes of trauma more complex, than such a theory can incorporate. Herman asserts that the 'victim', rather than giving up, will watch, scan, and observe her environment before and during any interaction, and that the 'victim' believes (through her experiences, whether justified or not) that she is always under scrutiny, and expects retaliation for her actions and behaviour. In relation to the work of Kurz (1987), healthcare professionals are perceiving the presenting woman's behaviour in isolation. By not acknowledging domestic violence as a primary diagnosis they are misinterpreting women's behaviour:

Some theorists have mistakenly applied the concept of 'learned helplessness' to the situation of battered women and other chronically traumatized people. Such concepts tend to portray the victim as simply defeated or apathetic, whereas in fact a much livelier and more complex inner struggle is usually taking place. In most cases the victim has not given up. But she has learned that every action will be watched, that most actions will be thwarted, and that she will pay dearly for failure. (Herman, 1992a, pp 90–1)

This assertion suggests that the behaviour displayed by women who have experienced domestic violence, identified as a stigmatising quality by medical staff, is perfectly acceptable and indeed 'normal' within the context of the battered woman's experiences. Rather than being 'evasive', they are reacting to a domestically violent situation which makes their behaviour a justifiable response. Failure to diagnose domestic violence as a primary factor will lead ultimately to such behaviour being considered 'abnormal' in some way, as opposed to being perceived as a valid and 'healthy' response to traumatic experiences. The prescription of tranquillisers and antidepressants only serves to label such women's behaviour deviant, and fails to incorporate domestic violence as a social problem which affects the experiences, realities, psyches, and physical bodies of women within society.

These problems have been addressed within theoretical work which has been conducted in Britain. Glass (1995) and Dobash and Dobash (1992) have examined the issues which affect women in relation to notions of 'victimhood'. The fact that both parties address the issue of 'victimhood' in relation to both the 'battered woman syndrome' and notions of 'learned helplessness' is particularly interesting. Dobash and Dobash (1992) suggest that although discrepancies arise when looking at domestic violence and health within both a North American and British context (particularly in relation to concepts of therapy and mental health), a therapeutic theme can be located in much of the theory surrounding domestic violence. This ultimately informs the way women who have experienced domestic violence are perceived within the medical interaction. This perception is not reduced within the Dobashes' analysis to the medical profession. It also includes critiques of social work practice and other social agencies through their use of therapeutic models of intervention. They suggest that the result of a therapeutic society and its influence on researching and understanding domestic violence is the individualisation of a social problem. They perceive the concepts of 'learned helplessness' and the 'battered spouse syndrome' as representative of such individualising processes which require the creation of individual women as 'passive', 'sick' and 'powerless'. While they believe that such perceptions of women who have experienced domestic violence may increase 'sympathetic tendencies', they suggest that it creates a negative public perception of the individuals involved. Again, this paradox can be clearly identified in the practice of the medical staff observed in the empirical research identified earlier. Their use of stereotypes, relating to women as passive, sick, powerless, vague, unhelpful and evasive, enables them to treat some women while excluding others through the mechanisms of the 'sick role' as a form of social control. On an individual level, this results in perceived 'good' women receiving treatment while so-called 'bad' women are being denied the same treatment. On a wider sociopolitical level, such practice, it could be suggested, results in the perpetuation of gendered, racist and economic power relations. This view is also held by Glass (1995), who suggests that the requirement to fulfil a specified role, in relation to the experience of domestic violence, renders women 'powerless' if they are required to become 'true victims'. Such a position subsequently locates women who have experienced domestic violence who do not display expected 'victim'-related behaviour as unworthy of help. Glass (1995) extends the occurrence of such paradoxes to the gendered expectations of women more generally:

> ... we are brought up to believe that women are the centre of the family and that in nearly all cultures it's women's responsibility to keep the family unit together. Not trying or failing to do so isn't only a sign of failure as a woman, but has the effect of 'unwomaning' – removing both her female essence and substance – and therefore rendering such a woman non-existent. (Glass, 1995, p 47)

The research examined earlier does not uncover why medical staff attributed stigmatising qualities to 'some' women who had experienced domestic violence and not others (beyond the existence of certain vaguely defined behaviours). It is therefore important to examine socially defined gender expectations as a possible determinant in the categorisation of women who have experienced domestic violence. Another important aspect of this problem is the perceptions of women who have experienced domestic violence. Much of the literature around domestic violence fails to adequately incorporate the experiences and perceptions of women who experience domestic violence, but this is not a criticism applicable to the work of Glass (1995). She bases her book, and the arguments within it, on the experiences and 'expertise' of women. The result is that theories of 'learned helplessness' are not always applicable to women who have experienced domestic violence. Such women do not automatically lose their own identities and subjectivity to a concept of victimage, despite the requirement to fit such roles in order to gain help. Glass demonstrates the ingenuity and reflexivity of women who find themselves in domestically violent relationships:

> "There was a lot of resistance about putting any form of label like that: battered woman, battered wife; my husband's domestically violent, he is a violent person; he's abusing me, he's misusing his power; and all the rest of it, all those sorts of labels. There was tremendous resistance to putting that label on me because I didn't want to wear it. Also it seemed false because when you were at work, you were up, together one hundred per cent and OK. So it was like you were a part-time battered wife. You were doing it job share." (Samantha, in Glass, 1995, p 60)

The above quotation and the assertions made by Glass generally, demonstrate how the holistic nature of theories of 'learned helplessness' are not particularly useful for women who are actually experiencing domestic violence. A notion of 'victimhood' does not fit easily into a concept of their own selves. It can therefore be dangerous if such a position is adopted by professionals (Loseke and Cahill, 1984; Glass, 1995) in order for them to understand the dynamics of the intimate relationship within which violence is present:

> Determining worthiness varies from culture to culture, country to country. Purity and innocence are most often used as indicators, but they are defined and weighted differently in different places. Nevertheless, though definitions may vary, each society seems to have a clear notion of what it means to behave like a 'real' victim. For a woman, this usually means being a passive, pathetic, pleading wretch. Assertiveness and self-possession are generally looked on with suspicion. A convincing female victim puts herself in the position of needing to be helped. To reject that begging role suggests wanting to take control, to make one's own decisions, to be free to live one's own life. (Glass, 1995, pp 183-4)

Because the wider experiences of self are important to our understanding of domestic violence, and therefore of its impact on health, the research on which this book is based considers the subjective experiences of the research participants[2].

Asking 'the' question: "Why doesn't she leave?"

The overriding focus of Glass' (1995) analysis of domestic violence and the power dynamics inherent within professional intervention ultimately undermines the nature of the questions which academics and other professionals ask. This critique is conducive to that of Loseke and Cahill (1984) who, in the process of challenging interventions by academic researchers, question why so many hypotheses concern themselves with 'why women stay within violent relationships' when such a question is flawed:

> By asking why battered women stay, the experts implicitly define leaving one's mate as the normative response to the experience of wife assault. Staying, on the other hand, is implicitly defined as deviant, an act 'which is perceived as violating expectations' ... once experts identify a woman as battered, normative expectations regarding marital stability are reversed. (Loseke and Cahill, 1984, p 297)

The types of questions which researchers (among others) ask construct the reality within which expectations about women who have experienced domestic violence are themselves constructed. Producing a notion that women who experience domestic violence should leave violent relationships, when there already exists a very powerful social discourse which advocates that women should keep relationships and families very firmly together, adds to those cultural myths which allow individuals both personally and professionally within all agencies to perceive women within violent relationships as in some way deviant or stigmatised in themselves. Such a position does not consider the impact of relationship breakdowns, whether domestic violence is involved or not (Vaughan, 1994).

> Staff members feel sympathetic towards women who say they are taking action to leave a violent relationship. (Kurz, 1987, p 73)

The quotation above reiterates the problems associated with asking specific questions by locating the negative responses of healthcare professionals within the expectation that women should leave violent and abusive partners. Perceptions of domestic violence patients are important, therefore, as are expectations about the behaviour of such patients.

This chapter has introduced literature which considers a number of theories relevant to a discussion of domestic violence and health. It has also examined empirical evidence from North America which has investigated this issue in depth. The research on which this book is based is contextualised within that work. The following chapters offer a detailed examination of British healthcare professionals' responses to domestic violence. There are occasions when similarities to the North American literature are evident, and also examples where the specific dynamics of the British health system make comparison difficult. In order to adhere to a feminist epistemological standpoint, the results of this research begin with a section concerned with the responses of British women who have themselves experienced domestic violence. Subsequent sections address health practitioners' responses to a number of concerns raised by these women and the literature above.

Notes

[1] For example, Leeds Inter-Agency Project, Derby Domestic Violence Action Group, Hammersmith and Fulham Inter-Agency Project.

[2] Due to the focused nature of this text, readers specifically interested in issues of subjectivity are referred elsewhere. For a discussion of the impact of domestic violence (and health) on the subjectivity of the participants, see Williamson (1999).

Part One:
Domestic violence patients speak out

The following three chapters are based on the experiences of women who have experienced domestic violence (stage one participants). They are intended to contextualise the health interaction within the experience of domestic violence and wider help-seeking activities. As such, they address: the impact of physical and non-physical injuries; a variety of treatment experiences; views of the health interaction; and wider experiences of help seeking. It is on the testimonies of these women that Chapters Six to Ten, which relate to responses from health practitioners, should be considered. The chapters in this section are important because they describe in detail how women who experience domestic violence interpret the professional response of the health practitioners they encounter. They also address issues relating to specific types of injury and therefore offer health professionals an understanding of the types of injuries women who experience domestic violence are subjected to. In relation to non–physical injuries, and issues relating to self and identity, the following three chapters also contextualise the participating women's wider interpretations of the responses of 'others' to domestic violence.

A large proportion of the oral history narratives conducted with the participating women focused on how they perceived themselves in relation to the domestic violence they had experienced and the help-seeking processes they engaged in (for a more detailed discussion of the research methodology, see Williamson, 1999). This book is concerned specifically with the interaction which occurs between women who have experienced domestic violence and healthcare professionals, and as such there is not the room to examine in depth the subjective histories of the participating women. It was important, however, to contextualise the impact of domestic violence in the participating women's subjectivity, as it was within the context of domestic violence itself that the health interaction took place. How they felt about themselves, the abuse they experienced and the wider help-seeking processes they engaged in constituted a large proportion of the interviews on which this book is based. Various issues emerged within these interviews including: self–blame; self-denial; the unreality of an abusive situation; contradictions of abuse; internalised anger; silence; dislike of confrontations and conflict;

fear; triggers to change; re-socialisation as part of the recovery process; the relationships between women who experience domestic violence; issues about male attention; power; suicide; and finally, issues around reproduction. It is not possible to examine all of these issues within this book and readers are directed elsewhere (Williamson, 1999) for a more detailed examination of issues relating to self, identity and subjectivity.

THREE

Physical and non-physical injuries

This chapter addresses the issues of both physical and non-physical injuries which the participating women sustained as a result of domestic violence. Making a distinction between physical and non-physical injuries proved important in relation to the response of health practitioners as well as the women from stage one. Just as definitions of violence and abuse can be problematic, so too do women who experience domestic violence feel these contradictions. This is compounded by abuse, which has a non-physical health impact and results in injuries which cannot be seen either by the participating women or 'others'.

Physical injuries

This section of Chapter Three is intended to illustrate the types of domestic violence-related injuries which women present to healthcare professionals. Out of the 10 women who participated in this research, eight had experienced physical abuse at the hands of an intimate male partner. While Jemima and Emma recalled only one physically abusive incident, the remaining six women described experiencing physical violence consistently throughout their relationships. In particular, Iris, Helena, Amy, Brenda and Carol (predominantly older women participants) described increasingly violent physical attacks which resulted in an escalation in the seriousness of their injuries. This finding is in keeping with previous research which suggests that violence escalates over time as the abusive relationship moves through a cycle of abuse[1] which repeats itself:

> Most of this violence, such as slapping and pushing, could be considered minor in the sense of having a low probability of causing an injury that needs medical attention (Stets and Straus, 1990). However, evidence shows that a proportion of these cases can escalate to severe acts of violence (Feld and Straus, 1990). (Aldarondo and Straus, 1994, p 431)

Only Debbie and Francis had not experienced physical abuse as adults. Four of the women, Amy, Brenda, Carol and Iris, had experienced physical sexual abuse within their domestically violent relationships. By identifying the abuse that the participating women experienced we can observe that the majority did experience physical abuse:

> "... the next day he'd look at me and my face would be out here and I'd have a black eye and a split lip." (Carol)

> "... he knee-ed me in the ribs four or five times, and he broke three of them and cracked one and I had a lovely sort of knee indentation down one side, well I don't know if you've ever broken a rib? But it effectively paralyses you ... well I think he must have realised that he'd done something reasonably serious and he backed off. Well I was just lying there, I couldn't move and breathing was difficult too." (Iris)

> "I fell on the floor, and I had concrete marks on my neck and grab marks on my arms and I mean if it had ended there I wouldn't have felt like I'd been beaten up but he had his hands round my neck." (Jemima)

The extracts displayed above give examples of the types of frequently recurring injuries which the participating women sustained as a result of domestic violence. Bruised[2] eyes and split lips were common to all the women who had experienced physical abuse, as were grab marks on either the upper arms or wrists. Less frequent and comparatively more serious (in terms of health implications) injuries included broken ribs (Iris), knife wounds (Carol, Amy), strangulation (Carol, Amy and Jemima) and long-term injuries to the eyes (through the frequency of receiving bruised eyes) (Carol).

> "[He had] a knife, and I put my arm to protect myself and it went through, and a friend of mine took me to the hospital." (Carol)

> "... I'd lose consciousness, they'd come and take me, and I'd just wake up in the hospital. The second time, I was very close to death 'cause I'd lost, he'd squeezed all my glands back and they'd all swollen up, like and all the oxygen wasn't getting to me, and they said if I didn't get enough oxygen I'd be brain damaged but ... that's life." (Carol)

The extracts above highlight the types of more serious injuries the participants from stage one sustained as a result of domestic violence. Carol's statement at the end of the latter extract also illustrates that such injuries are not perceived as uncommon within a history of abuse. Indeed, it has been suggested (Walker, 1979; Pence and Paymar, 1986; Herman, 1992a, 1992b) that women, as well as perpetrators, will understate the seriousness of the physical violence they experience.

Other studies have produced similar findings.

Box 2: Physical injuries

A sample of 57 women had sustained the following physical injuries: permanent eye damage, broken ribs (two), had been head-butted, punched in the head, choked, broken teeth, dislocated nose, head injury, bruising, broken nose (two), broken jaw (two), fractured skull, cracked ribs, knocked unconscious, stitches in the mouth, broken finger, black eye, split head, prolasped womb, ruptured eardrums, rape (five), attempted rape, miscarriage (two), premature birth and split mouth. (McWilliams and McKiernan, 1993)

Box 3: Physical injuries

Stanko et al also identified similar physical injuries and found within their study, which included reported injuries sustained by women as recorded within a GP waiting room survey, that 24% had suffered bruising anywhere on body, 16% cuts, bruises or marks on the face, 13% black eye, 12% cuts anywhere on body, 11% lost/broken tooth/split lip, 10% blackout/ unconsciousness, 9% bleeding on face/body/arms/legs, 6% sickness or vomiting, 6% sprained wrist or ankle, 5% broken nose, jaw or cheekbone, 3% burst eardrum or deafness, 2% burns anywhere on the body, 2% broken arm, leg or ribs, 2% miscarriage, and finally 2% of their survey experienced internal injuries. (Stanko et al, 1998)

Box 4: Physical injuries

Research from North America also identified similar injuries within a study which examined the types of injuries sustained by a group of 25 women who identified their injuries, within a medical setting, as being caused by domestic violence: 24% sustained abrasions/lacerations, 52% contusion/soft tissue injury, 16% a fracture/sprain/strain, and 8% a puncture/rupture. This particular study also identified the location of injuries and found that the majority, 36%, were aimed at the face/head/neck area, 28% were spread among multiple locations, 16% within extremities, 8% the genitalia, and 4% of injuries directed towards the chest/abdomen and back/buttocks. (Varvaro and Lasko, 1993)

By contextualising the findings of the research on which this book is based with those from other studies, we can observe that there are frequently recurring injuries which result from physical domestic violence. It is also apparent from the previous examination of the numbers of women who access medical help that they often access such help for frequently occurring physical injuries. There is no question that healthcare professionals are proficient at identifying and treating physical injuries such as those identified above. However, the issue of importance here is whether such injuries are treated within the context of domestic violence. This issue will be addressed further in the following chapters. In relation to frequently occurring injuries, however, the participating women also discussed instances where they administered their own treatments and/or refrained from accessing medical assistance. Very little has been written examining the informal networks of health provision which women who experience domestic violence access specifically for the treatment of injuries:

> "Oh yeah, there were times maybe if I just had a black eye or maybe a couple of bruises it's not really worth it, after I'd had about the third time I'd had the black eye that's when my mum said I think you should go to the hospital because I started to have problems with my left eye and she felt that my sight was going to be ... y'know that it was going to cause me problems later on in life, so I remember going up to the hospital I think it was the third or fourth occasion, they said there was some damage." (Carol)

Carol's experience shows that there were instances where she did not access medical assistance because she 'didn't think it was worth it'. Carol's mother was a nurse, as was Amy, and Brenda's abusive partner. In all these cases the women accessed informal help for their frequently occurring injuries, which in Carol's case resulted in the onset of long-term health problems. The reasons why women access informal health assistance will be examined shortly; however, one of the consistent reasons why the participating women avoided contact with healthcare professionals related to previous negative experiences. As the above discussion illustrates, the consequences of not accessing medical help are problematic in relation to frequently occurring injuries as well as more serious ones.

Finally, in relation to frequently recurring physical injuries, three of the participating women, Carol, Amy and Helena, all experienced violence during their pregnancies. This constitutes 50% of the participating women who had (biological) children. As well as discussing the domestic violence which she was subjected to, Amy also discussed how her experience of domestic violence generally impacted on her reproductive choices. Amy described how she had had a secret abortion, a traumatic and lonely experience (on account of her partner's Catholicism), because she did not want to bring another child into the abusive relationship. Conception was as a result of sexual assault. This illustrates how the impact of domestic violence on women's reproductive choices is actually much wider and more complex than the issue of violence within pregnancy:

> "He'd think nothing of hitting a pregnant woman, he'd think nothing
> of it because in the early days I used to think when I was pregnant,
> well at least he isn't really going to hurt me but I was very lucky I
> think that he didn't actually cause any damage to any of them, but at
> the same time, there were times I used to have to go to hospital, for
> false labour or once the waters was broken, at the front or the back,
> but the traumatic side of it is there." (Carol)

As a specific medical area of concern in relation to domestic violence, prenatal clinics and services have received much attention from other researchers. Injuries caused to both the mother and fetus as a direct result of domestic violence include premature birth, low birth weight and miscarriage (Webster et al, 1994; Chez, 1994; Denham, 1995; Norton et al, 1995; Schornstein, 1997). This body of research suggests that physical violence can begin and/or escalate during pregnancy (Webster et al, 1994). In a study conducted by Webster et al (1994) the types of injuries sustained during pregnancy were compared, within a sample of women who acknowledged experiencing domestic violence, to injuries sustained while not pregnant. The results of this study illustrate that gynaecological injury was reported as occurring "only when pregnant" by seven of the participating women[3], compared to two women who sustained such injuries "only when not pregnant". Similar results were found in relation to assaults towards internal organs during pregnancy (Webster et al, 1994). Due to the fact that violence may begin during pregnancy, the impact of violence on the fetus and therefore on the process of pregnancy, and also on account of the fact that prenatal services relate specifically to women-only services, issues of screening for domestic violence during pregnancy have been debated by a number of researchers and professional bodies (Webster et al, 1994; Chez, 1994; Denham, 1995; Norton et al, 1995; Schornstein, 1997; Friend et al, 1998). All of the research identified above illustrates that prenatal (and termination) health services are an important medical setting, and one within which the issue of domestic violence and health has already made an impact. As only one of the participating healthcare professionals in the current study was located specifically within prenatal services, the issue of violence within pregnancy is not a considerable aspect of this research. In relation to the clinical experience of this particular participant, however, violence within pregnancy will be readdressed in Chapter Eight.

Long-term health implications

It became apparent in the interviews with the participating women that there were a number of long-term health implications resulting from the physical violence they had been subjected to. In particular, the experiences of Carol demonstrated how repeated minor injuries can themselves cause long-term health problems:

> "I jumped up because he thought I was gonna pass out like I normally do, but by this time my nose and face were a mess, there was blood everywhere, he'd fractured my cheek bone, and he'd given me a black eye but he'd also burst one of the veins underneath, now and again I still have this pain in my eye, which again, I went to casualty, they sorted me out, I told them what had happened, but they gave me some treatment I was supposed to keep up, some cream and stuff to go on my eye, which I was never able to keep up, which I was supposed to go back for regular checkups on my eye, and I was never able to do that again, because he [the abuser] said I was wasting time." (Carol)

This extract demonstrates how the causes of an injury, whether of social origin or not, can effectively prevent the adequate treatment of that injury. This is a very serious issue which has massive implications for the use of resources and the long-term health of women who experience domestic violence. It is extremely unlikely that injuries with organic causes would be prescribed a treatment option which did not take into account the cause of the injury. Helena also had experience of the long-term impact of physical violence, as the following extract illustrates:

"I mean at that point he had bitten my leg so badly that I had marks on my legs for two years afterwards, he sank his teeth into my calf, he was pulling my hair out and pushing my head against a wall y'know, but I'd fallen down and he just fell on top of me and he bit me." (Helena)

As both of these examples demonstrate, it is important that healthcare professionals identify the cause of injury, in order to ensure that the treatments offered take into account the wider implications of living in a domestically violent relationship. These findings add impetus to those researchers (Bograd, 1982; Stark and Flitcraft, 1982; Klingbeil and Boyd, 1984; Klingbeil, 1986), identified in Chapter Two, who have challenged the misdiagnosis of domestic violence and the use of secondary rather than primary diagnosis. Again, this issue will be re-examined in Chapters Eight and Nine in relation to the clinical experiences of the stage two participants.

Non-physical injuries and psychosomatic symptoms

From the initial interviews with women who had experienced domestic violence it became apparent that, while physical injuries caused by physical abuse and violence were obviously relevant within a discussion of the health implications of domestic violence, women identify quite clearly the psychological effects of such abuse. Seven of the participating women had attempted suicide, four on multiple occasions[4]. In addition to actual suicide attempts (or para-suicidal activity), all 10 of the participating women had had contact with mental health services of one kind or another. These services included counsellors (both private and statutory), psychiatric services (frequently following para-suicidal activity), and psychologists. All of the participating women described their experiences of psychological and emotional abuse, and all attributed the mental health problems they had experienced to their domestically violent relationships.

The following interview extracts refer to psychosomatic complaints as described and identified by stage one participants:

"The denial has to come to an end one day whether physically her body will give her that ... because that's what's happened to me physically. I didn't realise just how things can take over." (Debbie)

This first extract, relating to non-physical injuries, is important because it demonstrates an awareness by Debbie that ignoring psychological problems will result in physical, psychosomatic illness and complaints. This breaking down of the mind/body distinction is clearly relevant when examining a professional practice which has such distinctions as the basis of its professional discourse. It also implies that taking an holistic/person-led approach to health and well-being is pertinent in cases where injuries are caused by domestic violence.

> "Because of all the trauma of the battering and stuff I couldn't eat because I was all yucky inside so I lost a lot of weight." (Emma)

> "I still have problems sleeping ... I get this knot in my stomach still I know every time, he used to come down, I always used to get this knot in my stomach, like anxious y'know and what's gonna happen and if he's in a good mood." (Carol)

These interview extracts acknowledge the symptoms of food and sleep disturbance as psychosomatic symptoms of domestic violence. These symptoms relate directly to issues of anxiety and depression, subjectivity and self-harm. The gendered prevalence of eating disorders (Wolf, 1991) is relevant here, as are the implications and functions of eating disorders for the individual involved. On a simplistic level, eating disorders frequently related to anxiety levels and stress experienced by the participating women as a result of negotiating a violent and abusive relationship. Eating disorders have also, however, been associated with self-harm and mutilation (Favazza, 1996), which raises specific questions about the health interaction in light of the seriousness of such widespread symptoms. Acknowledging the important relationship between eating disorders and control enables us to examine the actions of the participating women in relation to the subjective wounds women experience to their self-identity within a domestically violent relationship. Cross (1993) states that eating disorders, as well as self-cutting, represent "attempts to own the body, to perceive it as self (not other), known (not uncharted and unpredictable), and impenetrable (not invaded or controlled from the outside)" (Favazza, 1996, p 51). The implications of eating disorders will be examined shortly, in relation to other forms of 'destructive' behaviour demonstrated by women who experience domestic violence. However, the importance of basic bodily functions in relation to issues of control should not be underestimated:

Loathing an item of food, a piece of filth, waste, or dung. The spasms and vomiting that protect me. The repugnance, the retching that thrusts me to the side and turns me away from defilement, sewage, and muck. The shame of compromise, of being in the middle of treachery. The fascinated start that leads me toward and separates me from them. Food loathing is perhaps the most elementary and most archaic form of abjection. (Kristeva, 1982, p 2)

The quotation above refers to the importance of the body in relation to the possibilities of placing oneself as a 'subject' in relation to others. The impact of violence and abuse has very serious non-physical ramifications for the participating women and again raises questions about a medical discourse which differentiates between the mind and body in order to formulate biomedical/wound-led responses to ill health. It would be very difficult, for example, to differentiate between the impact of physical and psychological abuse when both appear to manifest themselves physically and psychologically as injuries sustained by the patient.

"... but there were very tell tale signs that would involve that, things would be, I'd start to not be able to eat, I felt sick all the time, I would be sleeping all the time, and certain habits would start, I'd start twitching and develop a habit where I'd like scratch the tops of my arms, I'd squeeze spots, scratch off. I would sit on the toilet in the middle of the night, scratching at goose bumps until they'd bleed, I just couldn't leave my arms alone, and I would like, be quite destructive to myself." (Frances)

Frances identifies her preoccupation with specific areas of her skin as part of a wider range of psychosomatic injuries she sustained within a psychologically abusive relationship. The significance of this particular psychosomatic manifestation is documented within literature concerned with self-harm more generally (Favazza, 1996):

Some neurotic persons persistently excoriate their skin by digging into it with their fingertips. They tend to focus their gouging on insignificant bumps or minor irregularities on their skin. Once such a focus is found, the individual experiences mounting tension, which is temporarily alleviated by scratching and removing the irregularity. Such individuals often try not to scratch but eventually succumb to tension. The persistent scratching has been interpreted psychodynamically as an attempt to express repressed rage toward authority figures and as a mechanism for ridding the body of badness and contamination. (Favazza, 1996, pp 148-9)

Frances identifies that certain symptoms which manifest themselves physically are related to her mental state, and act as signposts for her own management of such conditions. She also identifies that, while her symptoms were not representative of a serious psychological illness, she did suffer psychologically in relation to her sense of self:

> Traumatic events call into question basic human relationships. They breach the attachments of family, friendship, love, and community. They shatter the construction of the self that is formed and sustained in relation to others. They undermine the belief systems that give meaning to human experience. They violate the victim's faith in a natural or divine order and cast the victim into a state of existential crisis. (Herman, 1992a, p 51)

As with the discussion of eating disorders earlier, self-harm represents the exertion of power and control over the body, albeit damaging, in order to negotiate psychological relationships within the self. In relation to domestic violence, these symptoms relate to anxiety and depression, as well as the psychosomatic manifestation of psychological trauma:

> "... it was sort of like, I know what schizophrenia really is but it's like sort of the carry-on version of schizophrenia it's like being two people." (Frances)

Frances' comments above are particularly important as they are well documented within psychological literature relating to 'victims' of domestic violence (Walker, 1979, 1989, 1991; Post, 1980; Ferraro and Johnson, 1983; Carmen et al, 1984; Tuan, 1984; Herman, 1992a, 1992b; Worrel and Reiner, 1992; Kornblit, 1994; Saunders, 1994; Stark and Flitcraft, 1995, 1996; Hudson-Allez, 1997). In relation to borderline personality disorders, which can be found within the analysis of a "complex post-traumatic stress disorder" (Walker, 1991; Herman, 1992a, 1992b), the symptoms displayed by women experiencing domestic violence are often confused by healthcare professionals (Carmen et al, 1984) with the symptoms of multiple personality disorder or schizophrenia. Rather than the symptoms above being manifestations of such serious psychological illnesses, the physical and non-physical injuries experienced by the participating women have to be considered in relation to the effects of domestic violence.

Para-suicide

As the following extracts demonstrate, para-suicide is a very serious health issue in relation to the experience of domestic violence. As mentioned earlier, seven of the participating women had attempted suicide, four on multiple occasions:

> "I tried to commit suicide ... I didn't have any kind of what I'd have called real meaningful support, it was just a case of a pat on the shoulder, are you doing alright, and then leave." (Debbie)

> "You'd think they'd have something like that in central London, ten years ago y'know, obviously the problem ... she just called me a stupid little girl, I wanted to kill her, I wanted to just throw the bucket over her ... full of tar, puckies, and paracetamols floating in the top. I just thought well how flaming wonderful, y'know I've made a stand, I've tried to just shout here the only way I can think of." (Emma)

Both Debbie's and Emma's experiences of healthcare professionals following a suicide attempt represent how women's para-suicidal activity is often interpreted. While the second incident happened a number of years ago, and it could be argued that healthcare professionals are now more aware of the dynamics of para-suicidal activity, Emma found that the response she received negated the possibility of discussing the origins of her injury:

> "I ended up having a really bad breakdown, and one of these doctors came out, and he just, because I'd withdraw into myself so much, I remember being there but not being there, I'd lost the use of my mouth and I was just slurring and hyperventilating, and I was just a mess, a complete and utter mess, and I just curled up into this ball and they said I'd had this post-traumatic stress or something that had happened, and then they prescribed me with Valium ... yeah ... and I thought well really all I need right now is someone to talk to. To just give me Valium, I mean even in that situation it would have been so easy for me to [kill myself], I had them for two days, I had them to just kind of calm me down, but after the two days it was

very important for me because I realised that it's quite dangerous if I get addicted to them, that it took such an enormous amount of strength, to actually say to myself, don't do this to yourself. Don't back down that easy, it's not just about you becoming monged out of your tree all the time, y'know you've got to try and find other help. It was on my own back again, and they didn't follow it through, they prescribed me with Valium and I would have thought that if they'd seen that person in that state of shock they'd at least have someone come round a couple of days later and talk to me about it." (Debbie)

The issues raised here relating to the prescription of antidepressant and tranquillising drugs will be examined in more detail in Chapter Four; however, these issues are particularly pertinent in relation to para-suicide. Debbie felt that the prescription of Valium was both dangerous and a way for healthcare professionals to intervene in relation to her symptoms without acknowledging the origins of her injuries. Debbie also refers, in the above extract, to issues of power and control. Debbie felt that Valium removed her control and her refusal to comply with the prescription she interprets as a powerful act of self:

"I had a breakdown, and I can remember saying to my mum, that something was happening to me, I said I don't know what it is but I'm not right, I can't cope, I wasn't eating, I went right down to seven stone, I was really thin, I couldn't eat, and this went on for a number of years, and I used to keep telling people that I'm not myself, in the meantime, I'm taking these overdoses, even ... one day, even when I was speaking to my doctor, and I'd taken the overdose and he said are you going to do it again, this was on, I think it was the third time, and he said are you going to do it again, and I said if it's the only way I can escape yes, with that he said to me, I think you're having a breakdown, I said well I could have told you that months ago, and I went home and I was and I thought no, I can't deal with this, and so one morning after another violent beating I got up and I went down to [the] mental health hospital, I went in and I sat in there and I refused to leave until somebody saw me because I thought everything I've been going through within this relationship for the past 15 years of my life, at the time it was 14, the last 14 years of my life, and I said I need help, they got this doctor to come down and see me and he prescribed antidepressants for me, and I still said no I'm not going, I don't feel well enough to go home and be in charge of my children and live with that man, this was about a year before I actually came here, and in the end because he was left to cope with the kids, and carting them from my mum's and y'know around to different people, and all he was concerned with was when am I gonna get out? What you looking for attention for now y'know, you're just looking for attention, anyway I was on this course of anti-depressants, and they made me very lethargic, very ... all it did to me was make things not a worry no more ... not a problem ... nothing was a problem, he could hit me, and he could kick me and I'd get up after and be like well that's the way things are ... I just felt really worn down, it gave me no life, no spirit, so I went back to the doctor, well it's not helping, I said I'm coming off them from my own free choice because at the end of the day I think it's something I'm living with, I've got to come to terms with it and sort out a way of getting out of ... and that's what I did." (Carol)

I have included a large extract from the initial interview with Carol, as her experience of mental health services is particularly important. While Carol had attempted suicide on a number of occasions (four at the time of the interview), her actions as illustrated in the above extract demonstrate a non-destructive attempt at receiving mental health services to counterbalance the psychological injuries she had sustained as a result of domestic violence. Ironically, Carol's attempt to take action resulted in her being prescribed antidepressant drugs which she described as making her feel 'lethargic'. While in some situations the prescription of drugs may be appropriate, in cases of mental illness and/or within specific times of anguish and crisis, where the presenting woman may be taking action and accessing help for the first time, prescribing drugs (which dull the senses) only serves to reinforce the presenting woman's vulnerability and powerlessness. In all of the above extracts the participating women felt that they were not heard and that their extreme actions went unacknowledged.

Examining the relationship between para-suicide and the other examples of self-harm demonstrated in the above extracts, it is reasonable to suggest that women who experience domestic violence and who subsequently attempt suicide do so out of a will to live (Maris, 1971). Taking into account the injuries to self which domestic violence causes, the need to assert control within the self is a genuine one, expressed by the majority of women participating in this research. Considering the importance of para-suicidal and self-harming activity within this process, it is even more alarming when healthcare professionals do not take seriously the needs of women which lead them to take such drastic and self-defeating actions:

> This state of psychological degradation is reversible. During the course of their captivity, victims frequently describe alternating between periods of submission and more active resistance. The second, irreversible stage in the breaking of a person is reached when the victim loses the will to live. This is not the same thing as becoming suicidal: people in captivity live constantly with the fantasy of suicide, and occasional suicide attempts are not inconsistent with a general determination to survive. (Herman, 1992a, p 85)

The above quotation clearly illustrates how para-suicide relates to issues of power and control. Already, in the testimonies of the participating women, we can observe how they were indeed, at times of crisis, negotiating issues of power and control in relation to both the physical and psychological abuse they had experienced. Issues of control, however, were not divorced by the participating women from their help-seeking activities. In their interactions with healthcare professionals, the participating women were frustrated when they did not feel in control, when they felt that the interaction was being conducted without their collaboration, and when the professional did not take the domestically violent origins of their injuries and actions into account. The following chapter explores these treatment experiences in more depth.

Notes

[1] The cycle of abuse theory identifies the processes of tension building, battering and a honeymoon phase within the abusive relationship. For examples, see Dutton and Painter (1981) and Pence and Paymar (1986).

[2] While 'black eyes' is a commonly used phrase many black and Asian women find this phrase offensive and/or inappropriate and thus 'bruised eyes' will be used as an alternative.

[3] Total number of women within the sample, including those who had not experienced domestic violence, was 301.

[4] Amy had attempted suicide three times, Debbie twice, Brenda "several" times, and Carol four times.

FOUR

Treatment experiences

As was addressed in the previous chapter, seven of the participating women accessed accident and emergency departments for help during the course of their abusive relationships, and all 10 approached their general practitioners for help and/or treatment in relation to physical and/or non-physical injuries. This chapter will examine in more detail how the participating women experienced those interactions, what types of treatment alternatives they were offered, and what types of treatments they wanted. The following extracts demonstrate how the health interaction itself contributes to a woman's understanding of the abusive relationship she is experiencing and the wider help–seeking processes she accesses.

Validation of experiences and 'a sympathetic ear'

"... they prescribed me with Valium ... yeah ... and I thought well really all I need right now is someone to talk to." (Debbie)

"... they made me feel awful, I mean if I'd have got someone just for five minutes to say am I going mad, is this what real life is about, y'know, he's saying things to me and making me feel bad, is this right? I just wanted someone to verify what I was saying and to say no, it's not your fault, it's ok, that's all I wanted." (Emma)

Both of the above extracts are important because they relate to interactions which occurred as a result of para–suicidal activity. Both the extract from Debbie (also displayed in full in the previous section) and the extract from Emma illustrate instances where the participating women were particularly vulnerable and suicidal and when they wanted to have their experiences heard and validated through the appropriation of the sick role. Both of the women above had attempted suicide, and therefore located themselves within the biomedical discourse, for validation of subjective experiences which were occurring outside of it. The responses which Debbie and Emma received are consistent with a biomedical/wound–led model approach to mental health disorders. It could be suggested, therefore, that without holistic/person-led appropriation of the sick role, women who experience domestic violence may feel that in order to have their experiences validated they must resort to locating themselves within a biomedical model of health where their injuries are taken seriously. The irony, however, is that the appropriation of the sick role often excludes injuries including para-suicidal activity (Jeffery, 1979).

Both extracts demonstrate that the participating women do not simply want a 'sympathetic ear' which is neutral to the origins of their injuries, but that in order to counterbalance the effects of the abuse they have experienced they require healthcare professionals who will take a proactive stance and position which, while not judgmental towards the patient, help the patient to understand the reality of the situation she finds herself in. It has been suggested (Walker, 1979, 1989, 1991; Herman, 1992a, 1992b; Gondolf, 1998) that women who experience domestic violence do not understand the neutrality of the healthcare professional, due to their heightened awareness caused by the domestically violent situation:

"The only time they asked me out right [about domestic violence] was when he stabbed me." (Carol)

"I remember an instance shortly after that where I was in hospital and the nurses were very good because they just asked me very simple straightforward questions where all I had to do was say yes or no, but at school it was a little bit more different where I had to try and explain and ... I had never been in a position where I could have ever verbalised what was going on at home before, and I can't recall the words I must have said, but I can recall the sheer fear of what I was trying to say, there was a lot of fear." (Debbie)

Both the above extracts relate to contradictions inherent in communication between patients and healthcare professionals. The second extract, from an interview with Debbie, is particularly interesting, as she describes an event where the nurses she encountered asked her questions which required a 'yes' or 'no' answer. Debbie recalls that being able to answer 'yes' or 'no' reduced her fear at having to verbalise (and therefore acknowledge) what was happening to her. While women may want to talk to healthcare professionals, they may also be reluctant to verbalise their abuse, which suggests that a 'listening' approach will only be effective if the healthcare professional is aware of the sensitive nature of domestic violence and the problems patients have in verbalising such experiences despite a desire to do so. The issue of communication between patients, and examples of specific questions to both elicit information from individual patients and as part of a wider screening process, will be discussed in Chapter Thirteen, in relation to specific training tools and clinical resources.

Blaming women and 'other women'

It is essential that any interaction between women who experience domestic violence and healthcare professionals does not perpetuate the conditions of the abusive relationship itself. The following extract demonstrates how Helena was angry when a nurse implied that she had provoked the violence she had experienced:

> "... a ... nurse said to me, 'What did you do to upset him?' and I said, 'What do you mean what did I do to upset him? I didn't do anything', she said, 'Y'know you must have done something to upset him', and I said, 'Well if you call living normally', well I said something like that. I was absolutely outraged by this but y'know she said, 'You have to keep him calm', she said 'men don't do this unless women upset them', and I thought, what the fucking hell is she talking about y'know, women are, here am I just sort of going, I think something had happened, I think I was at work and I was a bit late or I hadn't picked the child up and I'd asked him to, y'know one of these things that's a trigger for him but seems perfectly normal and when you look back at it it's absolutely normal, and he just laid into me." (Helena)

The issues raised within the extract above are synonymous with testimonies of other women who have experienced domestic violence, in relation to their interactions with healthcare professionals and other statutory bodies (Pahl, 1985; McGibbon et al, 1989; Hague and Malos, 1993; McWilliams and McKiernan, 1993; Glass, 1995). Healthcare professionals clearly need to address their own feelings about domestic violence, evident within the extract above, in order to offer advice or listen to women in a way which does not perpetuate the abusive social discourse of domestic violence which blames women for the abuse they experience.

The extract also raises issues in relation to the gender of healthcare professionals, in that it is a female nurse's actions which Helena is describing. In relation to health visitors in particular, it has been suggested that the social policing function of female healthcare professionals undermines female solidarity (Riessman, 1983) within the health interaction. It is legitimate to question why the nurse Helena encountered felt she could say the things she did within a health encounter where she was the professional and Helena the patient who required treatment. In this particular example, the nurse is perpetuating patriarchal assumptions about the responsibility of individual women to manage men and their violence. This was introduced in relation to cultural myths in Chapter Two (Bograd, 1982). While it would be difficult to extrapolate a general explanation from Helena's interaction with this one nurse, it could also be suggested that this particular nurse was attributing blame in order to identify Helena as another woman, as different from herself and therefore 'other'. This would be supported by theorists (Dworkin, 1983) who have examined the relationships which women have with one another within a patriarchal social structure. The conflict between feminist advocates and the nursing professions is also acknowledged by Campbell (1992) who suggests that initial skepticism by advocates relates to the paternalistic attitude of many nurses.

Information and advice

In conjunction with the space to talk about their experiences, women often require information and advice, which they may only be able to access safely through healthcare professionals whose consultations are confidential:

> "I used to think about getting out, I mean now I can look back and think god, y'know how could I have put up with it, why didn't I known about these help lines and these places beforehand or why couldn't someone have given me the information, instead of just leave, leave, y'know? If I'd have been able to have gotten out of the situation maybe five, six years ago, my life would've been a lot better, but I think the length of time that I stayed within that environment has seriously damaged me." (Carol)

This treatment option is important, as some women felt that they didn't want direct 'help' from the health interaction, but more choices, which can only be offered if healthcare professionals have information about domestic violence and the diverse range of voluntary and statutory services which exist locally. Considering the diversity of women's help-seeking activities (McGibbon et al, 1989; McWilliams and McKiernan, 1993), rather than prescribing advice about limited services it is important that healthcare professionals offer patient-orientated treatment options and have adequate knowledge about a range of services, advice and information.

The above extract also demonstrates the changing expectations of patients within the medical/health encounter. Research (Salmon et al, 1994) suggests that general practitioners are particularly poor at detecting patients' intentions within the medical encounter. This is due to a number of factors, not least that patients change their intentions and requirements in relation to specific health-related problems. In relation to psychological problems, for example, Salmon et al (1994) found that patients wanted 'support' and not medical treatments or information. Due to differences in predicting expectations, such patients were often subjected to inappropriate medical investigations which culminated in patient dissatisfaction, non-compliance, and inappropriate treatment and referrals:

> "I think if I'd have been in the situation where those services were in place, I still would have never have recognised that.... I think in the early days I don't think I would have recognised that I needed help ... for some strange reason ... I think maybe that's got a lot to do with pride ... I'm only actually coming out of it and accepting that I still need help to deal with it." (Debbie)

> "... that's the only time that they said, well how did you get this wound, and I said that y'know [he stabbed me] and she said that really she should report it to the police y'know but that if I didn't want her to then she wouldn't." (Carol)

The above extracts from interviews with the participating women demonstrate how difficult it is to intervene and 'help' a woman who presents with a domestic violence-related injury. While not contacting the police when you are genuinely concerned about a patient must be extremely frustrating, there are other non-statutory services which could have been accessed in both these cases[1]. It is important for healthcare professionals to understand the need women who have experienced domestic violence have to control the situation they are in. Due to the effects of abuse and violence, many women feel out of control and have little power within their intimate relationships. Any help-seeking activity is contextualised, therefore, within the wider experience of domestic violence. It is essential that the medical encounter does not perpetuate feelings of powerlessness and lack of control. Research already suggests that professionals generally find it frustrating when women do not leave a domestically violent situation (Glass, 1995; Stark and Flitcraft, 1996; Schornstein, 1997). This paradox is theoretically exacerbated within a medical encounter if the treatment model being adhered to has implicit within it a concept of health absolutism. While a woman is still in danger, offering her advice which assumes she can leave such a situation will perpetuate a woman's powerlessness and lack of control and will ultimately result in further isolation. Isolation is itself a method which abusers utilise to control their female partners. When women are made to feel responsible for the actions of their abusers, this method of control is extended from the abuser to wider social interactions. Healthcare professionals need to ensure that their interactions with women who experience domestic violence do not indirectly mirror the tactics used by perpetrators to control the behaviour of their partners.

Being 'struck off'

It became apparent from interviews with the women participating in stage one that some doctors found the frustrations of dealing with domestic violence-related non-physical injuries beyond their professional expertise:

> "And when your doctor turned round and, who I'd have thought were the first person who could have put you in contact with help, when even he says he couldn't find a solution because basically it's a case of well get your act together ... or else, and because we couldn't because we didn't know how to, we were struck off the list. Y'know so that rejection was the biggest blow that I could have experienced." (Debbie)

Both Debbie and Brenda were struck off from a general practice after suicide attempts relating to domestic violence. As Debbie describes above, the effects of this rejection on her self-esteem were insurmountable and did nothing in assisting her to make positive choices relating to her experiences of violence and abuse. This issue raises many questions about the patient/professional relationship and the responsibility of each within such a relationship. Shifts towards more holistic/person-led models of healthcare have resulted in contradictions in the changing power relations which exist between patients and professionals within the medical encounter (Donahue and McGuire, 1995; Peters et al, 1998). As the extracts above demonstrate, the responsibility which doctors have for their patients' medical well-being results in the location of practitioners within a paradox. This paradox positions them, rather than patients, as consumers within the medical encounter (Sharma, 1994). The holistic medical model and market-driven conceptualisation of healthcare may result in reconceptualisations of power within the medical encounter. However, it must also be acknowledged that, as professionals, doctors in particular remain in a position where they can withdraw their medical knowledge and clinical expertise from particular patients. Thus, these individuals are deemed to have failed in their responsibility as patients (Finerman and Bennett, 1995). The examples given in the above extracts undermine theories which suggest that power within the medical encounter has shifted through a move towards holistic and community-based concepts of healthcare. In both these cases, practitioners have removed their services through the use of holistic concepts of health, by suggesting that patients can be denied treatment where they abdicate responsibility for their own health and well-being. This is despite the fact that the presenting patients have been injured as a result of the actions of others.

Lack of advocacy

The participating women's criticisms of healthcare professionals' treatment of domestic violence-related injuries were most often related to a lack of advocacy and follow-up intervention. The lack of ongoing advocacy was perceived, by the women from stage one, as representative of a lack of support and understanding about domestic violence. This lack of ongoing support was considered to represent the underlying apathy of healthcare professionals towards their patients experiencing domestic violence:

"... they encourage you to do that [referral to crisis mental health services], you make a big step to do that and it is sometimes hard, well it was for me that initial step, and in all that time I never once got a letter asking how I was, not a doctors letter, it was never on my files, it was a major cry for help, I could have died and yet no one in the medical profession, no one heard it." (Emma)

"I would have thought that if they'd seen that person in that state of shock they'd at least have someone come round a couple of days later and talk to me about it. Nobody following it through for me, nobody rang up, y'know I just thought the system isn't geared up to sort of ongoing help, it's here's your tablets, take two or three of these a day, and come back to us when you feel like you want some more and I thought that's not what I want...." (Debbie)

"I think maybe my view or outlook may have been negative but I would have still have wanted somebody to have been committed that they're going to see this through with you to the very end. No matter what you say, no matter, and that I would have appreciated, somebody who wouldn't have backed off, y'know, because to me, it would have been, it would have changed my cynicism." (Debbie)

There is obviously an issue of resources in the above concerns raised by the women participating in stage one. Ongoing support and advocacy is expensive and is not a problem limited to interventions by healthcare professionals. It is, however, a problem which faces healthcare professionals alongside other statutory and voluntary services which are accessed by women presenting with domestic violence-related injuries. The relevance of inter-agency collaborations and initiatives will be discussed in more detail later; however, there is a need for healthcare professionals to identify whether follow-up intervention is appropriate in particular cases. In practical terms, health advocacy would involve ensuring that follow-up letters would not put the presenting patient in more danger, and if so, raising the issue when the woman next presented in the surgery. The majority of the participating women were particularly critical of the medical profession when they perceived that they had made an attempt to seek help and it was not heard or acted on. While this lack of advocacy can be perceived in relation to the lack of continuity in healthcare generally (Oakley, 1981), it is clearly recognised as a specific problem by the presenting women.

Counselling

The issue of counselling arose in the interviews with all of the participating women. Half (five) of the women had had counselling, although the type and duration differed considerably, from one single session to long-term specialised counselling services within a feminist framework:

"I wouldn't like to say that all counselling was positive because I've met some that aren't, and again it's about quality, I've met some really bad counsellors and I don't think I've met some really good counsellors apart from the woman who I had. I think counselling what it does is it gives you a comfortable space to work things out but it's like working things out for myself, if somebody started telling me how it was, I don't think I'd find that quite productive." (Debbie)

"... but even now, when I came here I used to say to the people in the refuge that I needed counselling." (Carol)

In Carol's experience she would have liked counselling, but it was not a service she was offered by any of the professional or voluntary agencies she accessed for help. Within the voluntary sector, lack of outreach support is a recognised problem which has resulted in many refuges establishing befriending services and outreach support for their ex-refuge residents (Hague et al, 1996)[2]. As with most services, lack of funding often prevents this type of intervention, which does not specifically address crisis service provision. Debbie's own experience of counselling was good, although even within such services she perceived the need to remain in control as an important part of her 'recovery' process. Debbie also points out that not all counselling is appropriate, and that there are 'good' and 'bad' professionals and professional practices:

"Y'know I'm articulate, I'm able to work things out for myself ... it's just I needed to have some kind of counselling, to kind of have some kind of constant support, not only for myself, but also when I was coming to the house all the time, I was seeing that there were problems with the family as well and it's just all too much and I thought anybody who knows anything would have understood that. It was like nobody ever addressed it and I just could not in the end face having to repeat my story over and over again and I thought sod this, I'm just going to go out there and do what I can, so it was only by that point that I realised that the only person I can count on is myself." (Debbie)

"... she paid for me because she realised that it was an important part of my self-development, so y'know every week I'd go for a session, and she'd pay for it, so that helped because I couldn't afford to go, and that's half of the trap, money, if you want help you have to pay for it, and I didn't have the financial means to do that." (Debbie)

Another important aspect of the counselling process, as part of a range of treatment options utilised within the medical/health interaction, is resources. In Debbie's second extract above, she identifies how receiving financial support was the only way she could access counselling on a long-term basis. Debbie also, in the first extract, identifies how a lack of continuity left her feeling disillusioned with such interventions. As with criticisms which relate to the lack of continuity and advocacy in interactions with healthcare professionals, continuity within counselling is also important. Many of the participating women found counselling useful when it resulted in them being able to access wider support networks in order to reduce their isolation. Where limited counselling services were engaged in, the participating women sometimes interpreted the lack of continuity as apathy on the part of the counsellor.

The issue of counselling, in particular the role of the community psychiatric nurse (CPN), emerged as important in the study conducted by McWilliams and McKiernan (1995). They found that five of the women in their sample were currently receiving CPN services, and that the CPNs themselves recognised the impact of domestic violence-related issues on their overall caseloads (McWilliams and McKiernan, 1995). It is generally accepted, however, that adequate counselling services, in terms of resources, do not exist nationally (Harwin, 1997, p 142). The participating women's experiences of counselling differed significantly, therefore, in relation to the range of professionals they had to access in order to receive such services. This issue requires more detailed research in order to identify how counselling is accessed and utilised, by women who experience domestic violence and by professionals alike.

Prescription drugs

Despite the concerns about counselling raised above, counselling does represent a move away from the prescription of antidepressant and tranquillising drugs. As mentioned above, Debbie explained how she felt that she had been prescribed drugs in place of having her experiences validated. She was not alone in expressing this issue, as four of the participating women explicitly commented on how they had been prescribed drugs:

> "When I went to the psychiatrist which I told you about earlier, he asked me if I ever had suicidal thoughts and I said yes I did, I had thought about it, at the end of the interview he gave me a prescription,

and he gave me enough drugs to kill an elephant, whether or not he was trying to save the health service money I don't know. I got them home and thought this guy's loonier than I am and I threw them down the toilet, I had sleeping pills, antidepressants, shit loads of stuff, four or five different stuff in a big bag like a supermarket carrier, go home and kill yourself basically...." (Iris)

"So I went through that process and ... at some point the doctors kicked in and tried to prescribe me some tablets but I was crap at taking them, because I didn't mind the behavioural therapy because I was in control but I didn't want to take the tablets." (Frances)

"... they got this doctor to come down and see me and he prescribed antidepressants for me, and I still said no I'm not going, I don't feel well enough to go home and be in charge of my children and live with that man ... in the end because he was left to cope with the kids ... all he was concerned with was when am I gonna get out? What you looking for attention for now y'know, you're just looking for attention, anyway I was on this course of antidepressants, and they made me very lethargic, very ... all it did to me was make things not a worry no more ... not a problem ... nothing was a problem, he could hit me, and he could kick me and I'd get up after and be like well that's the way things are.... I just felt really worn down, it gave me no life, no spirit, so I went back to the doctor, well it's not helping, I said I'm coming of them from my own free choice because at the end of the day I think it's something I'm living with, I've got to come to terms with it and sort out a way of getting out of ... and that's what I did...." (Carol)

The importance of moving away from drug-dependent interventions is clearly illustrated in the extracts above. Iris is extremely critical of the way in which she was prescribed drugs at a time when she could have used them to attempt suicide. A further issue is that managing the effects of domestic violence with antidepressants, without the appropriate support and recognition of domestic violence as the cause of the injury (whether physical or non-physical), results in the problem being defined in terms of the mental health of the presenting woman and not the behaviour of her male partner (Klingbeil and Boyd, 1984; Goldberg and Tomlanovich, 1984). In Carol's case she found that the drugs enabled her to cope with the violence, by effectively cutting off her senses, but did not assist her in making positive choices about the violent relationship she was in. Another important issue in the extracts above is asserted by Frances in relation to control. This issue has emerged already, but the patient can ignore or deny the treatment given in medical interventions if they do not feel they are in control of their help-seeking processes. The use of counselling as a treatment option, while problematic in some cases, is a positive move away from the prescription of drugs which, as the extracts above demonstrate, can be damaging to a woman's sense of safety, place her in a position where she can act out para-suicidal tendencies, and reinforce a lack of control within the help-seeking process.

Self-medication

The concept that women who experience domestic violence may not access medical assistance for frequently recurring injuries was introduced in the previous chapter. This was made possible by self-treatment, utilising friends and relatives, and known healthcare professionals:

> "… the day before I'd taken an overdose and my mum, she was a nurse and she'd put a funnel down my throat and put salt water so I'd vomited most of the tablets so I only had a little bit still left in me, because they was sleeping tablets I was very lethargic." (Carol)

> "I'd made quite a number of attempts on my life within that fifteen year span that I think that by then my mum was getting a bit fed up to be honest like I said she worked there and most of the people in casualty knew her and she sort of … that's what she gave me at the time, a funnel down my throat and poured all this salt water down it and I had to drink that and I vomited up most of the tablets anyway." (Carol)

The two extracts above refer to one specific incident which Carol experienced following one of her suicide attempts. This is a particularly extreme case of self-medication, and also implicates a trained health professional, but is one of a number of incidents where the participating women accessed informal health services, friends, and relatives for a variety of reasons. Reasons included their own and/or others' embarrassment, as well as the perception that the presenting women were not worthy of health services. Rather than access services which had previously resulted in negative experiences, the participating women used friends and family to obtain the healthcare they required. This use of an informal health economy is not itself unproblematic, as it has been suggested (Wallman and Baker, 1996) that the responses of others, whether health professionals or not, combine cultural, economic and clinical factors beyond more formal medical/health encounters[3]. It is clear that the impact of social constructions of domestic violence as a phenomenon is not restricted to medical encounters, but influences the options, medical and non-medical, which women have available to them. It is for this reason that Chapter Five will situate the medical interaction which this research has focused on within the wider help-seeking processes which women access.

Another issue in the above extracts is the frequency with which healthcare professionals themselves are implicated in informal help seeking. The relationships between healthcare professionals' personal and professional responsibilities to deal with domestic violence-related injuries are evident here. The responsibility of healthcare professionals to address this relationship has been examined in literature from North America (Campbell, 1992; Doner, 1994; McAfee, 1994; McDowell, 1994; Butler, 1995) which suggests that healthcare professionals have a moral imperative to deal with the issue of domestic violence as social citizens, in conjunction with their professional responsibilities. In the above extracts, the differentiation which exists between these positions is evident. It was also evident in the responses of the healthcare professionals, which will be examined in Chapter Six, where only three of the second stage participants referred to their social responsibility to deal with domestic violence outside their clinical practice.

Documentation

The medical record is important in relation to domestic violence, as very often it may be necessary to prove the occurrence of physical violence and injury at a later date, in criminal proceedings. Many of the participating women assumed that, because they had received medical treatment for physical injuries, their medical records would document years of violence and abuse which could be utilised to prosecute the perpetrator of their violence at a later date:

> "Yeah, I know when I went to court one time, and I was always told that they kept records, but they didn't have much records, they only went back a year or so, I thought they would keep that, even though I didn't tell them, how I got the injury ... sometimes I told them, a lot of the time, I'd always tell someone, if I didn't tell the doctor I'd

tell the nurse, I'd always tell somebody, but, when I actually went to court and this had been after ten years of it, there was only about a year on record." (Carol)

The above extract illustrates how Carol was disappointed that her medical history did not document the catalogue of serious and frequently recurring injuries she suffered as a result of domestic violence. Again, research from North America clearly identifies documentation as the most important intervention a healthcare professional can make in relation to the majority of domestic violence-related injuries they are presented with (Hadley, 1992; Vararo and Lasko, 1993; Stark and Flitcraft, 1996; Schornstein, 1997).

Another very important issue relates to the knowledge which patients have regarding their own medical records. Although patients can have access to this information, the participating women were often unaware of this fact. The result was that they did not know whether they would be able to call on their medical records as evidence during criminal proceedings or whether the healthcare professionals with whom they had interacted were aware and had recorded domestic violence as the cause of injury.

> "I'd have told them yeah ... because I still wonder, those letters, surely those, would they be on my medical records? That's what I was just thinking, I had this at the doctor's the other day actually.... I had to carry my medical records from one end to the other and I was so tempted to just stop off and go into the toilets and sit and read it.... I was really tempted you know because I was thinking I wonder what I'd find in it, I wonder what ever happened to all those letters that were sent...." (Carol)

The assertion made in this extract is interesting, as the access which patients have to medical records was one of the reasons given by healthcare professionals as to their reluctance to explicitly record domestic violence on the medical record. The issue of documentation, which is clearly central to a medical encounter, also has implicit within it issues relating to disclosure, as discussed earlier.

Documentation is important, as it ensures that women's experiences are recorded. It can also act as a form of validation, in that healthcare professionals who record the domestic violence origins of an injury can explain to the patient the importance of doing so, which validates the woman's experiences. Further, documentation raises issues about screening for domestic violence and ensures that, if adequately recorded, future misdiagnoses may be avoided. Finally, documentation is particularly important for research, in order to identify the prevalence of domestic violence generally and in relation to specific professional practices; they can also be utilised to examine the personal and financial costs of domestic violence. The views and clinical experiences of the participating healthcare professionals in relation to documentation will be examined in Chapter Ten.

Generic examples of bad practice

"I suppose my feeling is that the medical profession should stop treating women as hysterical, I think that's a violence against them as well." (Helena)

"... they didn't really push you, because there were some nurses that said you should tell someone, you should tell your doctor, or you should leave [the relationship], or others who were just, after three or four times I think they just got fed up of seeing me, they'd print up something from the computer and realise I'd been there before and they were just ... [they'd] walk away ... shaking their heads." (Carol)

"... when I went with broken ribs and stuff they made no mention of a follow-up, or counselling, domestic violence unit, he didn't mention a thing, he left it, the onus was on me to deal with the situation to get out from under him and make sure it doesn't happen again. How? How do you make sure it doesn't happen again? You do what most women do and look for the trigger and you avoid them and you're nice to them. There was no back-up given to me and I presented with a reasonably serious injury, and I know a lot of women suffer horrendous injuries but it was back to me, it fucking shit my life up at the time." (Iris)

Helena was articulate in her belief that an inappropriate response to domestic violence by professionals within the health service was itself a form of violence against the presenting woman. Indeed, the concept of the medical encounter itself being part of the wider problem of domestic violence, abusive in and of itself, has been documented (Warshaw, 1994; Stark and Flitcraft, 1996; Schornstein, 1997). In this context, it is not surprising that Carol interpreted the actions of the nurses she encountered (whether accurate or not) as judgmental and dismissive of her situation. The reasons why nurses may feel freer to make social judgments about women presenting with domestic violence-related injuries was examined earlier, in relation to an experience which Helena recalled (p 49).

Another important issue concerns the gate-keeping process nurses must administer in order to ensure the smooth running of particular health services (specifically in secondary health provision). It is suggested (Byrne and Heyman,1997) that rather than nurses having poor communication with patients, they employ specific techniques in order to facilitate their specific and general responsibilities and in order to avoid difficult questions. The general responsibility which nurses have for the smooth running of a particular department often results in them carrying out the tasks of others, which leaves them less time to offer psychological and emotional support for the patients in their care. The implications of collaboration between nurses and doctors on patient care and the organisation of health provision will be examined again in Chapter Eleven. The way in which the dynamics of interactions between health professionals impacts on their ability to offer specific forms of care is nevertheless important.

Awareness of professional frustrations and constraints

The following extracts demonstrate that women who present with domestic violence-related injuries are often aware of the frustrations and constraints which influence the ability of healthcare professionals (and others) to deal with various issues, including domestic violence. The participating women were also aware of these frustrations prior to the medical encounter:

> "I think they should take an interest really.... I know they're understaffed and stuff these days but I think they should take an interest because you are their patient aren't you?" (Carol)

Carol's assertions demonstrate both an awareness of the problems facing healthcare professionals and a belief that women who experience domestic violence are patients too. Carol's use of a disclaimer at the end of the above extract is also evidence that, although she believes domestic violence 'victims' to be worthy of adequate treatment, she is aware that such patients may be differentiated from the general patient population:

"Unless they're a 40-year-old practitioner who knows your family or would be concerned if something untoward happened, but generally people are moving around all over the place and moving practices, they don't have family doctors like they used to anymore, I don't think you get that close relationship. I mean I used to go to this doctor and he delivered me, do y'know what I mean and anything untoward happen an' he'd be on the ball, not into domestic violence I suppose, the last time I saw him which was ten years ago he's probably never heard of it, he'd probably experienced it but there wasn't a label for it, any groups or agencies out there so, yeah, I think I feel sorry for them because I'm sure some of them would like to do more, I really do, but they don't want to scrape away the top surface because of what they're going to find underneath. There's so many problems that are occurring, weight loss, stress, anxiety, depression, there's an underlying problem and they're there to, they probably have got guidelines, and they're there to treat what they see." (Emma)

Emma is clearly aware of the constraints which frustrate healthcare professionals and which prevent them from dealing adequately with domestic violence-related injuries. In particular, Emma identifies psychosomatic and non-physical injuries as creating problems for healthcare professionals. She also identifies the importance of a biomedical/wound-led model of healthcare where she states that doctors simply 'treat what they see'. While this perspective is not advocated through specific guidelines, such a distinction is inherent in the medical paradigm. Emma also identifies changes in medical discourse where she differentiates between old style 'family doctors' and the less personal interaction which occurs when people change their doctors due to geographical mobility. This limits the possibilities for person-centred treatment available within the doctor–patient relationship. Despite identifying this difference, Emma contradicts herself by stating that her own general practitioner, who she identifies as a 'traditional' family doctor, was not aware that she had been experiencing domestic violence the last time she had seen him. It could be argued that Emma is actually attempting to understand a lack of medical response, despite her explanations being undermined by her own experiences within the medical encounter. This issue of the different types of doctor–patient relationship arose also in Carol's interview. Carol also had a family doctor, who she had known since childhood. Due to this, she felt embarrassed telling her general practitioner the cause of her domestic violence–related injuries:

> "He [family doctor] did, he asked me, at the time I was a bit embarrassed to say and 'cause he'd known me from birth like and was our family doctor, I didn't want to tell him." (Carol)

The above extracts are interesting, as they highlight how patients have reconceptualised their relationships with healthcare professionals, a shift which mirrors the changing relationship between biomedical and holistic models of healthcare (Douglas, 1994; Sharma, 1994; Kelner and Wellman, 1997; Peters et al, 1998). While the participating women accept that addressing issues such as domestic violence must be frustrating for healthcare professionals, acknowledging that a woman is the only person who can judge her safety is central to an approach which is catering to the patient's need. The 'health absolutism' (Gallagher and Ferrante, 1987) advocated to increase good health in patients is not appropriate to domestic violence, because in some cases remaining in the violent relationship may be a positive choice when one is fearful for one's life. There are clearly problems, however, where health absolutism is advocated for medicalised social problems which are beyond the control of the presenting women. Theorists (Douglas, 1994; Sharma, 1994; Kelner and Wellman, 1997; Peters et al, 1998) have problematised the shifts between biomedical and holistic models of healthcare by questioning the motives behind such moves. It has been suggested, for example, that "the personal *right* to take responsibility for one's own health is all too easily elided with the civic *duty* to take this responsibility" (Sharma, 1994, p 90). Evidence for a continuing shift towards holistic healthcare, and thus responsibilities, can be found within the government's recent White Paper, which advocates the evaluation and implementation of 'consumer' triage services in the form of telephone helplines (Wyatt, 1998). This move not only replaces doctors with trained medical nurses and new information technologies, but restricts access to health services by placing responsibility on the patient to utilise health services more effectively. This shift has inherent within it a number of contradictions, between a medical discourse with increasing social jurisdiction and measures intended to limit access to an increasingly overwhelmed profession (Southon and Braithwaite, 1998; Weale, 1998). The wider social and political implications of these developments relate to the emergence of the medical discourse and its position within an increasingly medicalised social discourse[4].

Communication breakdown within the health service

The participating women were concerned with what they considered to be a lack of communication between healthcare professionals within different medical services. This was considered particularly problematic with regards to information sent from casualty departments to general practitioners. This information, which is usually conveyed via a 'flimsy'[5], often went missing, was required to be delivered by the patients themselves, or was not responded to by the general practitioner. This particular communicative device was important in cases of para-suicide (which affected seven of the participating women):

> "Yeah, the doctor, he knew, he used to get the letters, every time you went to casualty they used to give you a letter to give to your doctor, but he never, not ever mentioned anything to me about it. I'd go back there for like other things but he'd never mention it." (Carol)

The criticism evident in the extract displayed above is aimed at a general practitioner for not responding to the 'flimsies' received from the accident and emergency department of the local hospital. This issue was raised by a number of the participating women, many of whom felt that this response represented a lack of concern with the issue of domestic violence and the patients themselves. These perceptions were particularly relevant to the communication between healthcare professionals, as the participating women believed that the documentation of their interactions would precipitate further action from other healthcare professionals. This issue of communication and collaboration, both between healthcare professionals and within an inter-agency context, will be addressed again, in Part Three of this text. While there are problems, including professional communication and documentation, which are specific to the medical profession, these issues also face other professional groups who are accessed as part of a range of help-seeking activities. In order to identify where professionals can learn from one another in relation to generic issues of bad practice, the following chapter considers wider inter-agency help seeking.

Notes

[1] The reasons why healthcare professionals may feel more comfortable referring to statutory professional agencies will be addressed in Chapter Twelve.

[2] Research is currently being conducted by Hilary Abrahams, University of Bristol, in this area; see also Kelly, 2000.

[3] The impact of the responses of 'others' on the subjectivity of women experiencing domestic violence is not addressed explicitly within this text; see Williamson (1999) for a more detailed discussion of this issue.

[4] For a more detailed discussion about the emergence of the medical discourse and the current contradictions facing it, see Williamson (1999).

[5] A flimsy is the method of documentation utilised within secondary health services.

FIVE

Wider experiences of help seeking

This research emerges from concerns (identified in Chapter One) that healthcare professionals are not adequately represented within inter-agency initiatives advocated by national government (Hague et al, 1996). As such, the role of other professionals, both in research about domestic violence and in professional practice, is important to the research on which this book is based. In relation to the participating healthcare professionals, the issue of inter-agency collaboration will be addressed in Chapter Twelve. In order to contextualise the stage one participants' experiences of domestic violence and help seeking, it was necessary to examine their experiences of interventions with other professional groups. This helped distinguish between general professional practice and clinical practice specific to the health professions, and also enabled examination of how the participants' experiences of health interactions were perceived and contextualised in relation to other professionals. The women who participated in the research identified a range of professionals with whom they had had contact. These included the police, the criminal justice system (including court welfare officers and solicitors), social services, teachers, and a range of voluntary service providers including refuges. This chapter examines the participating women's contact with statutory agencies only[1].

The police

The police are obviously one of the first points of call for a woman experiencing domestic violence. This intervention is usually related to specific incidents and crisis intervention. In many cases, the police will be called to a domestically violent situation by a third party: a neighbour or friend. The following extracts illustrate how women who have experienced domestic violence perceive the intervention they have had with the police within various contexts:

> "You see when I was younger and it used to get out of hand and I was in fear for my life which I was many a time, I used to call 'em out [the police], but I thought that's what you do, that it was okay to

do that, and I was more calling them to try and calm the situation or make him realise that somebody else knows what's happening." (Carol)

"... the only thing they [the police] concern themselves with is a statement, and if you don't give 'em a statement then they don't really want to pursue anything, they just say look 'If I come back out here you'll both be in trouble for breach of the peace'. At the time they'd say one of us has to go and they'd say 'If you have to come back, one of you leave the home for twenty-four hours and if you have to come back within twenty-four hours you'll be done for breach of the peace', so ... he ... obviously that's what he'd do, he'd go away, but he'd be back within a couple of hours, and then I'd be too scared to call 'em again, you know I didn't want to ... but on this occasion, the seventh occasion, this officer spent about three hours in the house with me doing a statement, and he [the perpetrator] wasn't supposed to come to the house, this was a Friday, and they'd told him not to come back to the house until the Monday, and they'd arrested him and kept him in the cells but obviously they had to release him after a couple of hours. Sunday he was on the phone giving me all this abuse, little did I know until I turned around while I was on the phone, that he was in the phone box, y'know, at the top of the road, and I could see him in the phone box, so I quickly put the phone down, rang up, apparently they were on another emergency, but three of them came away from this other emergency, and went looking for him, but they couldn't find him." (Carol)

The above extracts from Carol demonstrate how she perceived the police response and why she contacted them in the early stages of the abusive relationship she was in. Carol began with the impression that the police would assist her, an impression which changed through interactions with the police, who concerned themselves with 'obtaining a statement'. There has been much research focusing on the response of the police to domestic violence (Radford, 1987, 1992; Wilson and Daly, 1992) and much improvement in specific areas of the country, with the development of police domestic violence units (Hague et al, 1996). These experiences have also led to government police policies and innovative community-based police responses to domestic violence (Bridgeman and Hobbs, 1997; Plotnikoff and Woolfson, 1998; Hanmer et al, 1999; Kelly et al, 1999). Despite these initiatives, Carol clearly perceived that the officers she had contact with were more concerned with receiving a statement with which to prosecute the offender than to offer meaningful support, which is what she required. She also felt that the threat of prosecuting on the grounds of 'a breach of the peace' was directed to her as well as to the violent perpetrator. In Carol's case, she was, on a subsequent occasion, prosecuted for wasting police time.

The criminal justice system

If a woman decides to utilise the criminal justice system as part of her help-seeking process, the next step following intervention by the police is intervention within the legal system, through the courts:

> "... a couple of times I wanted to go to court, I wanted to take him to court, but it's very difficult when you're living in the same house as the person that you're going to court against so, its obvious that within, y'know before the court hearing date he would get me to drop the charges and unfortunately that's what happened and unfortunately it happened on seven occasions." (Carol)

Carol's extensive experience of the criminal justice system is particularly interesting as she identifies the strain and extra pressure which a court appearance for domestic violence places on what was an already violent and abusive relationship. Carol also discussed in her interview the reaction of the court usher, which was clearly one of frustration and little understanding of Carol's ongoing situation at home. While making professionals aware of these issues is not likely to stop the abuse of women happening, when they wish to prosecute their violent partners greater understanding would have enabled the court usher in Carol's case to offer her support and advice, rather than limit her future options. As has been mentioned, Carol was herself taken to court for wasting police time. With the greater inter-agency collaborations which exist at present (this situation is likely to change due to recent cuts in funding for such projects) in some geographical areas, and the more widespread training of professionals generally, it is not clear that this course of action would be taken now. The effects of this police action, however, demonstrate very clearly the ways in which women who are 'victims' of domestic violence are implicated as deviant, not only socially and culturally (Glass, 1995; Lloyd, 1995), but in this case criminally also.

Solicitors play an important role in inter-agency collaborations, although again this group was nationally recognised for its lack of representation (Hague et al, 1996). This is unfortunate, as not only do solicitors have a role as legal advocates within the inter-agency process generally, but they also have a role as advisors in the women's help-seeking activities. Very few of the healthcare professionals interviewed for this particular research referred to the role of solicitors as advisors, nor as being able to offer legal and criminal advice as an alternative to the police. The following extract is from one of the women from stage one, and refers to the way in which she experienced help seeking when she approached a solicitor:

> "This other occasion when I did actually go to a solicitor and got a decree nisi, in court, the solicitor in the run up to it, I can hardly remember anything about it but I remember this one thing, and he said 'So how long have you been married?' and I said that and he said 'When did the beatings start?' and I told him that and he said 'and do you enjoy it?' And that, exactly the same feeling I had towards this nurse and I said 'What do you mean do I enjoy it?' and he said 'Some women do', and I said 'Either you or them are mad', I mean I wasn't really a feminist at the time, all I knew was it was the most appallingly ridiculous question which somehow was said in such a way that these people believed it, had a view of women that women actually incite men to beat them up or a view of women that means that men believe that women enjoy it. I couldn't believe it and he said 'Well y'know'. Of course I didn't enjoy it, and he well 'Yes I suppose not, you're getting out after two years, some women y'know', they think that they do enjoy it because women put up with it, 'Y'know I have women sitting here y'know they've been in marriages for thirty years', and I was still struggling with this and I don't think I answered him at all but in reflection the answer that should have been was, if they have had as much trouble as I have had trying to get away from this man I'm not surprised that women sit in front of you after thirty years because they wouldn't have been ... nobody takes in a woman who's got a violent husband." (Helena)

Helena's comments are common in relation not just to solicitors, but to professionals in general. Many professionals hold stereotypical beliefs about women generally, and women who have experienced domestic violence in particular. These preconceived ideas are not surprising, considering the way in which women are labelled deviant, culturally and as we have seen criminally, despite being 'the victim' of a legally defined crime.

Social services

Social services very often have a role to play in the help-seeking activities of women living in domestically violent relationships, particularly when children are involved. Although many of the participating healthcare professionals made a distinction between issues of domestic violence and child abuse, there are studies which suggest that there may be a connection between the two, either directly or indirectly (Herman, 1992a; Wolfe and Korsch, 1994; Zuckerman et al, 1995). Indeed, the participating women from stage one clearly identified in the interviews the devastating effects that domestic violence had on their children, whether that was through the extension of violence towards the children or through witnessing violence and abuse committed towards the women themselves.

> "Social services came down and got me a car, and I went down and got the kids." (Carol)

Clearly, where children are involved social services have an important role to play within the inter-agency process. In the case of women who do not have children, the significance of social services as a source of help was minimal; it was surprising, however, how many healthcare professionals referred to social services as the main professional agency they would contact in domestic violence cases they were presented with. Recent research (Mullender et al, 2000) has examined in detail the impact of domestic violence on children, both generally and in relation to children who experience domestic abuse.

Teachers

None of the healthcare professionals identified teachers as an important resource in terms of information and support. If I had focused more specifically on issues of child protection and child abuse this may have been different. The role of teachers in the help-seeking activities of women experiencing domestic violence within a situation where children were present was significant:

> "They [the children] used to always tell me things and they could always talk to me but what I used to say was the effect that it was having on them, and the teachers, when I used to have to go see the teachers, 'cause he'd never go and see the teachers, unless he thought

I'd say something about an incident and he would make them think he was so intelligent and his children didn't suffer anything and he couldn't understand why they're throwing chairs around the room, why they're having these temper tantrums. I mean my eldest boy put a hole through a school wall, because he'd seen me beaten up the day before, he'd gone to school and some child had said just one little thing and, he just used to have these outbursts and the school were thinking this child's got something mentally wrong with him and I thought well I have to tell them some kind of background as to why he's got this problem, I knew he had a problem, but he would never acknowledge it up to this day, he won't still acknowledge any of his children. Even now, he's heard that I'm trying to get them counselled, he's totally against it, I think his fear is that he knows things are going to come out that he doesn't want to come out." (Carol)

"... it had been taken and noted by the PE teacher, that's how it started, because I wouldn't be allowed to do PE, I would be sent with a note all the time, and I'd be told to make excuses, y'know, you fell down the stairs, or somebody, I was told actually to say that somebody bullied me from another school. And I wasn't allowed to say how it really was. So when the PE teacher took note, that's how they got social services involved." (Debbie)

The impact of domestic violence on children is beyond the scope of this study; however, teachers and others involved in the care, education and health of children have a central role to play in domestic violence inter-agency initiatives (Mullender, 2000a). This collaboration is vital not only in relation to educating children and young people about the dynamics of violent and abusive relationships, addressing issues of power and control, and offering children support services themselves, but also in being able to assist women who access help through professionals who have contact with their children.

Notes

[1] For a discussion of the participants' concerns and experiences of voluntary sector organisations, see Williamson (1999).

Summary to Part One

A number of key points can be extrapolated from the participating women's experiences of domestic violence, which have been the focus of this section. These are summarised below. Many of these points also emerge in Part Two. The fact that both women who experience domestic violence and healthcare professionals themselves raised these issues is important. It suggests that better communication between patients and health practitioners could greatly improve the services women who experience domestic violence are offered. Better services to this group of patients, if combined with appropriate individual responses, would undoubtedly improve the health and well-being of health patients.

Box 5: Injuries

Taken from this small sample, domestic violence-related injuries included:

- Frequently recurring injuries, such as bruised eyes and bruising to upper arms and wrists.
- Serious injuries, including broken ribs, strangulation, weapon wounds and internal injuries.
- Violence during pregnancy to both mother and fetus (should be considered in relation to wider reproductive choices).
- Psychosomatic injuries: self-harming, eating and sleep disorders, anxiety, depression, and various components of the complex post-traumatic stress disorder.
- Para-suicidal activity.

Box 6: Treatment experiences

Key areas for consideration in relation to treatment options are:

- Women want validation of their experience and a 'sympathetic ear'. Patients may not disclose the origins of their injuries, which makes 'listening' problematic. Being 'neutral' should be avoided.

- Women often felt blamed. Professionals should offer a non-judgmental approach and not distinguish between women who experience domestic violence and 'other women'.

- Provide information and advice. Have an adequate knowledge of such information in order to be in a position to provide it.

- Consider the impact of striking a patient off a general practitioner's list where domestic violence may be an issue.

- Be aware of women's need for advocacy. This relates to validation, professional assistance and to general practical help.

- Always consider the role of counselling carefully. Never facilitate joint counselling.

- When prescribing drugs remember that women who experience domestic violence are more likely to engage in para-suicidal activity.

- Be aware that women can and do self-medicate. Consider your own responsibilities beyond the professional role. Many women are assisted in self-medication by trained health professionals.

- Always record domestic violence and explain to patients that they have access to such information. This is an easy way to empower women in their help seeking.

- Consider that women are aware of professional constraints and frustrations. This knowledge, culturally transmitted, influences their own sense of self-worth.

- Examine ways in which communication can be improved between healthcare professionals. This is particularly important in relation to para-suicidal activity. Women assume you talk to one another.

- Finally, women remember good, caring, non-judgmental and supportive healthcare professionals. Although the participating women may have only acted on these positive interactions years after their occurrence, the women remembered such experiences and the impact they had. The response of a caring healthcare professional can make a profound impact on a woman's choices and quality of life.

Box 7: Wider help seeking

The following is a list of professionals with whom the participating women had had some form of contact. Again, this list is extensive considering the small number of women included within this sample. A much wider and comprehensive range of professional bodies should be included within inter-agency initiatives, and health practitioners should be aware of the participation of other professionals.

- Education: teachers, education welfare officers.
- Criminal justice: police, court ushers, court welfare officers, probation officers, solicitors.
- Social services: social workers, community care workers, residential workers.
- Housing: housing officers, hostel workers.
- Voluntary sector services: women's refuges, women's centres, alcohol and drug services, mental health provision.

Part Two:
Clinicians' knowledge and clinical experience of domestic violence

The following five chapters are concerned with the responses of the participating healthcare professionals (stage two participants) to a number of qualitative questions relating to domestic violence. The first two chapters are specifically concerned with the knowledge which healthcare professionals have about domestic violence outside the health interaction which occurs between them and women experiencing domestic violence. These two chapters also consider how the participating healthcare professionals view domestic violence in relation to their professional roles generally, and begin to examine how they perceive both domestic violence and the domestic violence patient. Chapters Eight, Nine, and Ten examine the clinical knowledge which healthcare professionals have regarding a range of issues which emerged in Part One. This section will address the similarities and differences between the perceptions of both groups of participants. Also, where the responses of the participating healthcare professionals can be contextualised within data from the domestic violence and health questionnaire sample (Abbott and Williamson, 1999), this data will be included for discussion. This section demonstrates the views which health practitioners hold in relation to domestic violence and violence-related injuries. As such, it offers baseline data with which to examine improvements in practice which may occur as a result of recent policy initiatives.

SIX

Definitions of domestic violence, roles and responsibilities

This chapter focuses on definitions of domestic violence suggested by stage two participants. This question was asked to ascertain whether any of the healthcare professionals worked to guidelines or a strategic definition of domestic violence. All the stage two participants were asked "How would you define domestic violence?". Asking this question, in conjunction with questions about the general role of specific healthcare professionals, was intended to examine how participants located domestic violence within medical discourse, both theoretically and in relation to their clinical practice.

> "How would I define domestic violence? It's not something I've given a lot of thought to, to be honest." (Dr Quadir)

The extract above was not a common response, as the majority of healthcare professionals who participated in this research had clinical experience of domestic violence-related injuries, and it was an issue they had considered. In order to contextualise the issue of definitions of domestic violence within general health policy, all of the healthcare professionals who completed the domestic violence and health questionnaire (Abbott and Williamson, 1999) were asked if they worked to a formal policy when treating women who have experienced violence/cruelty from a male partner; 96.7% answered "no" to this question, with only 2.3% answering "yes". The discussions which take place in the following sections relate, therefore, to the definitions formulated individually by the participants and in response to policy-led discussions within the health professions generally. As recent policy initiatives and guidelines (DoH, 2000) have emerged in Britain since this research was conducted, this research also provides baseline comparative data on which to measure the impact of such guidelines.

Generic definitions of domestic violence

> "Obviously violence within the family, usually between partners, I
> hate to say husband and wife because in [specific town] [laugh]
> that's a dying institution…. I think it's something in the past that
> was brushed over was accepted as part and parcel of their [women's]
> role in society and accept that this was going to happen and I think
> people are now accepting this is not the case…. if I define domestic
> violence I wouldn't necessarily restrict that to physical violence which
> I think is one portion of it." (Dr Padden)

The interview extract raises several issues about definition. When asked
to define domestic violence, Dr Padden begins by questioning the
dynamics and structure of families within society. This issue emerged
in other stage two interviews, where healthcare professionals used their
definitions of domestic violence to identify those individuals who they
considered to be the perpetrators and the 'victims'. For example, Dr
Fagan stated that he had "not really treated any men to be honest but I
have treated homosexual partners who have come in with violence so
it is still domestic violence" (Dr Fagan)[1]. In relation to the identification
of 'victims' and perpetrators, Dr Gabb identifies the problematic nature
of domestic violence as a reference to violence between adults. Dr
Padden also identifies issues relating to different types of violence and
abuse, the historical context of domestic violence, and the social response
to domestic violence, in his definition above. These definitional
components will be examined individually within the following sections,
and in relation to similar issues raised by the other participants.

Differentiations in relation to age

> "You tend to think of it as adults, I mean I suppose technically
> speaking and from the definition I've given then age doesn't come
> into it but you tend to restrict it to consenting adults." (Dr Gabb)

This extract differentiates between domestic violence and child abuse, a
distinction which arose in definitions offered by health visitors in
particular. This differentiation was due to the heightened awareness
healthcare professionals have in relation to issues of child protection, as
identified in the 1989 Children's Act. All of the healthcare professionals
who were interviewed acknowledged that domestic violence does not
just occur between intimate partners who are married, but also between

cohabiting partners. Many also acknowledged that issues of elder abuse and child abuse could be incorporated within a definition of domestic violence, although in most cases they were more reluctant to incorporate child abuse than elder abuse. This illustrates how domestic violence is considered problematic due to the age of the 'perpetrators' and 'victims' involved. Yet all of the participating women who had children discussed at length how they perceived the domestic violence they had experienced to impact on their children, both through direct abuse and the witnessing of domestic violence itself. Various theorists have examined the impact of domestic violence on children (Hendricks-Matthews, 1993; Straus and Smith, 1993; Zuckerman et al, 1995; Hester and Radford, 1996; Hester et al, 1998; Mullender et al, 2000) and have questioned the adequacy of differentiating between the adult nature of domestic violence and the impact of such abuse on the family unit as a whole. In relation to the responsibility of professionals to deal with domestic violence, it is important that Area Child Protection Committees[2] discuss and take seriously the relationship between domestic violence and children. Their reluctance to make this connection is represented by the stage two participants' differentiation between violence against women and against children, and their responsibilities to deal with each.

Historical context of domestic violence

In the first extract from Dr Padden above (p 80) he locates domestic violence within an historical context and compares his perceptions of the current social response to domestic violence to women's historical acceptance of abuse. Including this historical consideration in a definition of domestic violence is interesting, as it suggests that the concept of domestic violence and its definitional value is itself socially, culturally and historically embedded. This involves shifting concepts of the private and public spheres[3], and the naming of domestic violence, both the act and process, by feminists in the 1970s. Researchers who have examined other professional groups have found that the notion that women 'accept' domestic violence is one reason given for a lack of intervention (Edwards, 1986). While Dr Padden identifies this 'acceptance' within a shifting social discourse, it is interesting that he includes this in his definition of domestic violence.

Physical versus non-physical abuse

Finally, Dr Padden acknowledges that restricting domestic violence to physical abuse is problematic.

> "Well any situation in which one or other partner feel that they are being physically threatened by the other. In some cases there are not actually marks to be seen. There is not actually real evidence of injury but there [has] clearly been the intent or the threat and people are frightened as a result." (Dr Fagan)

> "Well I think that I would define it in physical terms, although there are obviously cases where there is just psychological abuse. Domestic violence to me really means physical violence." (Dr Iannelli)

While both Dr Fagan and Dr Iannelli acknowledge the non-physical aspects of abusive relationships they perceive the importance of such abuse differently. Dr Iannelli clearly sees his role as a general practitioner as limited to physical abuse, which is extremely problematic. Fortunately, most healthcare professionals were willing to accept that domestic violence can take the form of physical, emotional, psychological and sexual abuse, although some of the respondents were more comfortable focusing on the physical and emotional aspects of abuse – areas where they perceived their own intervention as being most productive.

The general acceptance that domestic violence is a generic term to refer to violence and abuse within intimate heterosexual (and male homosexual) relationships supports the definition adopted for the purposes of this study. Although this research has focused specifically on the experiences of women who experience domestic violence perpetrated by their male intimate partners, the statistical predominance of this type of domestic violence was confirmed by the healthcare professionals' own experiences of treating predominantly female patients for such injuries.

Definitions of clinical roles in relation to domestic violence

Following questions designed to ascertain the general definitions of domestic violence utilised by healthcare professionals, none of whom worked to specific practice guidelines and/or definitions, I asked the stage two participants to define their roles as health providers, both generally and in relation to domestic violence. This was intended to identify how the participants perceived domestic violence to be located within medical discourse in relation to their clinical practice and professional roles. The responses to these questions were particularly interesting, as they outlined many of the barriers and frustrations which healthcare professionals perceive which prevent them from dealing adequately with a number of issues, including domestic violence. This demonstrates that before we even begin to examine the medical interaction itself, healthcare professionals perceive their interaction with women who present with domestic violence-related injuries as problematic:

> "I just tend to take it [domestic violence] in my stride really, I don't think that it is a specific problem anymore than sort of like diabetes or you know, it would be nice if it wasn't there but I do not find it a particular problem except when you, I mean some ladies they complain and say 'I am not staying with him' and then you go through all the recording of details about the case and then the next week they are back together again and, you know, they won't make any complaint against you know what is sometimes fairly vicious men.... But if the woman was willing to carry it on then I would support her." (Dr Iannelli)

Dr Iannelli begins the above extract with a statement comparing domestic violence-related injuries to other symptoms which he is presented with. He then contradicts himself by stating that "there isn't any particular problem with domestic violence ... except...". Already, through the use of a theoretical question about the role of healthcare professionals, this general practitioner is demonstrating preconceived ideas about how to deal with domestic violence through social and legal sanctions. Dr Iannelli also ends this extract by defining under what circumstances he would support a female patient experiencing domestic violence. Although he does not explicitly state that he would not support patients who do not leave abusive relationships, he clearly finds it frustrating when women do not leave their abusive partners:

> "I do sympathise, but I just haven't got the time because I do a lot of other things, [asthma] surgery, things like that, yeah it is very very frustrating. You see these people come through the door, you say 'next' and this woman comes in and you can tell straight away sometimes and think oh, 'it's going to be one of those' and your

art sinks because you want to help and you feel very frustrated ...
...d despite wanting to help you've also got a responsibility to other
people, patients waiting and to some extent you don't give them the
service they deserve." (Dr Padden)

The extract above also refers to the role of the general practitioner in
relation to domestic violence. Dr Padden admits that he finds treating
women who have experienced domestic violence frustrating, and that
before the patient even sits down he has called on a reserve of knowledge
about such patients in order to identify that such patients are frustrating.
This assertion is congruent with studies (Stimson, 1976) which suggest
that general practitioners have profiles of patients who they prefer to
treat.

> The least troublesome type of patient was defined as male, intelligent,
> employed and middle-class, with specific, easily treatable organic
> illness. The most troublesome patient was female, not employed,
> working-class, described vaguely as 'inadequate', and possessing diffuse
> symptoms of psychiatric illness that were difficult or impossible to
> diagnose and treat (Stimson, 1976). (Oakley, 1993, p 14)

This definition of the ideal patient includes not only demographic
characteristics of the patient but the type of injury or complaints they
present with. As illustrated in Part One, women who experience
domestic violence often have psychosomatic and/or psychiatric
symptoms resulting from domestic violence. It is exactly these types of
injuries which frustrate professionals in their clinical practice. It is in
relation to findings such as these that the way in which practitioners
define their roles and responsibilities is important:

> "The general practitioner's responsibilities and role is ever expanding
> and we just seem to be absorbing more and more and more ...
> community care beds disappearing and putting people back in the
> community, and we're having to look after them, mental health beds
> are virtually nonexistent and a lot of 'don't care' in the community
> happening and at the end of the day our time's being eaten away
> with less and less time for everything else, this [domestic violence] is
> just one of many things really." (Dr Padden)

In the extract from Dr Padden he admits that he does not give patients
experiencing domestic violence the treatment they deserve and explains

this by focusing on his responsibility to treat other patients and time restraints. As this quote above demonstrates, this can be located within the wider processes of medicalisation. Dr Padden is suggesting that domestic violence is one of many issues (particularly mental health issues in relation to care in the community) which utilise a large proportion of health service resources. He makes a distinction between issues which are being absorbed within the medical profession and 'everything else', for which there is less time. Dr Padden is therefore differentiating between valid medical complaints and those which prevent healthcare professionals from addressing valid complaints.

Non-medical practitioners' perceived roles in relation to domestic violence

So far the interview extracts have come solely from general practitioners. It is important to acknowledge that the relationships between healthcare professionals, in conjunction with the relationships which exist between patients and healthcare professionals, have elements of power inherent within them. For example, there is debate about the power dynamics inherent within the relationship between doctors and nurses. It has been suggested that the relationship between doctors and nurses can be contextualised within the concept of the 'doctor–nurse game model' identified by Stein (1967). This model suggested that nurses, while appearing submissive to the authority of doctors and physicians placed higher within the medical hierarchy, utilise non–verbal and 'cryptic' verbal cues to influence doctors while maintaining the hierarchy of healthcare professions (Hughes, 1988). This model and others like it (Freidson, 1970) have been challenged by researchers (Hughes, 1988; Svensson, 1996) who believe the relationship between doctors and nurses to be more complex and reciprocal than the 'game model' suggests. For example, Svensson (1996) suggests that a 'negotiated order perspective' is more appropriate to describe the inter-professional relationships between nurses and doctors, whose relationships have been affected by changing differentiations in status, women's position within society, and shifts in the biomedical orientation of healthcare itself (Svensson, 1996). While these theories differ in their perceptions of nurses' power within the doctor–nurse relationship, they all incorporate within them aspects of gendered power which, it could be suggested, mirror power relations beyond the medical profession. The ways in which gendered power is mediated within the medical hierarchy is particularly important in relation to this book, as we are examining the ways in which such power operates in wider society. Acknowledging that such power is also existent within the help-seeking structures which women access enables us to begin to challenge the constraints which face both patients and practitioners.

The power inherent within the medical hierarchy is also important in relation to the changing role of healthcare itself. The emergence of the medical profession has seen an increase in the medicalisation of various social problems. This has led to a current crisis, where the professionalism of certain groups within the medical hierarchy is inextricably linked to issues of medicalisation and, subsequently, de-medicalisation. The differentiation between the doctor and nurse roles has significant implications for the rewards and status accorded both groups, in that nurses are viewed as far lower on the medical hierarchy. Despite calls for the greater professionalisation of nursing, it has been suggested that, while professionalisation would help secure greater status for the work of nurses, it would not necessarily be women (the majority of nurses) who would benefit from such a process.

> For example, while only some eleven per cent of British hospital nurses are male, a disproportionate twenty-three per cent of senior posts within the hospital nursing service are held by men (MacGuire, 1980). (Oakley, 1993, p 6)

Even within professions in which women dominate in terms of numbers, their male colleagues are usurping the power women have by their over-representation in positions of authority. Due to the way in which the nursing profession is hierarchised, nurses have failed to successfully unionise as a profession, as the differentiation between nursing roles itself serves to divide women in terms of power, status and responsibilities (Oakley, 1993). This is not a necessarily bad thing. Having only precariously achieved the status associated with professionalisation, nursing, it has been suggested (Oakley, 1993), does not face the lack of confidence currently facing medics. Nurses are therefore in a position to challenge the over-medicalisation of health and to contribute effectively in the reconceptualisation of healthcare[4].

This discussion demonstrates how non-medical health practitioners are in a complex and potentially influential position regarding medicalised problems. Their views on domestic violence are therefore important, as are their perceptions about the non-medical role generally:

"It's difficult. I find it frustrating sometimes because it's such, about not being able to take themselves out of the situation, you find it very frustrating that you want to make things better, nurses always do, and they don't seem to want to or they don't seem to be able to and to keep visiting and to keep trying to support people with what decisions they make and you can get very frustrated with it because you think you've got the answer and you think you can ... 'if only you would leave him', if only they would, but they don't and they keep going back and keep letting the men back into their lives and I find that quite frustrating." (Ms Lacey)

The extract above, from a health visitor, reiterates the same frustrations which have already been expressed by general practitioners. It locates the professional frustrations which individuals feel within the social discourses which influence how women who experience domestic violence are perceived in wider society. As with the extract from Dr Iannelli (above), this extract focuses on the frustrations which are caused within domestic violence-related health interactions when a woman fails to leave a violent partner. The impact of such a focus was discussed in Chapter Two (Loseke and Cahill, 1984), in terms of the implications of choosing to ask why women stay rather than other pertinent questions. Clearly the healthcare professionals quoted here find the interstices between the medical and social discourses of domestic violence to be problematic which, due to their desire for women to leave violent and abusive relationships, results in further professional frustration.

Health professionals' perceptions of general roles and responsibilities

In conjunction with identifying their professional role in relation to domestic violence, I also asked the stage two participants to identify their professional role more generally:

"I don't even think GPs know what it is at the moment.... I see a number of changes, I've certainly experienced a lot of changes in the role of the GP and certainly having been looking at the GP and what's happened in healthcare over the last couple of centuries, it's interesting how the role of the doctor in society has ... altered ... when I qualified there was a distinct impression that medicine was crisis intervention and that patients came to us with problems and we sorted them out, now however there's quite a ... change in that we are being expected to be much more pro-active, health promotion, actually disease prevention and health education is much more on the agenda ... medical students have always looked at disease and how to sort of treat them once they've happened and now there's a great switch in emphasis. On top of that, not only is there a great shift in health prevention, health management, health education but also the ... GP as a businessman, y'know the sort of manager ... things like fund-holding ... we're always going to have something like that, so we're going to always have to manage our resources, not only clinical but it's going to have financial implications as well." (Dr Jabber)

The extract above is important, as it became apparent within interviews with general practitioners in particular that the way in which they perceived their professional role more generally was related to whether they perceived medicalised social issues as frustrating or not. Those professionals who located their medical practice within a shifting definition of medical discourse were less likely to find such change frustrating and more likely to admit when they were wrong, take advice from patients, offer patient-orientated healthcare, and were generally more aware of wider social issues and the manner in which they impacted on their professional responsibilities.

Just as the participating women from stage one identified changing concepts of health roles as important, and the general practitioner role in particular (Chapter Five), so too did three of the participating general practitioners:

"I think there's more of a levelling between the relationship, there's much more of a confidante, teacher, adviser, friend even, whatever role, before it was more pedestal. There's a practice not far away that its only in the last 10 years that he has left that he didn't even have a seat for the patient in the room, so y'know the patient stood up in the presence of the doctor ... and received a prescription and was in there for less than two minutes y'know, and one wonders about the quality of the consultation. But I think there's a move to sort of long, patients want to know, well, why are you doing that? Why do you think that? And there's an acceptance that I've found that if I've made a mistake and I say 'I'm sorry but I think it's happened because of X, Y, and Z', most patients, 99% of all patients, will say fine I can understand that, I can accept that. It's when people perceive that we're suddenly going back onto our white cloud or our ivory tower that they then think." [shrugs] (Dr Jabber)

This extract identifies changes within the doctor–patient relationship and locates those changes within shifts of power between both parties. Dr Jabber is describing what other doctors referred to as the 'Dr Finley' style of healthcare, where the professional status of the general practitioner precluded the possibility of a consultation based on the negotiation of power and knowledge within the health interaction. In relation to professional frustrations and constraints, Dr Jabber suggests that a move away from this style of practice enables him to interact more productively with patients on an equitable basis. He is aware, therefore, of the impact of his professional status on the perceptions of his patients. This issue is important in relation to a number of concerns raised by the participating women from stage one. First, domestic violence patients often need to feel in control of their help seeking. By locating the health interaction within a context which acknowledges the power and control of the practitioner, this relationship can be negotiated with the patient. Second, a number of stage one participants felt that health practitioners were judgmental about both them and their domestically violent situations. By understanding the power dynamics of the health interaction, practitioners can challenge not only practices, described above, which perpetuate the differentiation between professional and patient, but can also challenge the neutrality which such a position requires and which women find representative of apathy and disinterest.

In relation to the general roles and responsibilities of the participating non–medical health professionals, both health visitors and practice nurses perceived their roles to be shifting in relation to their relationships with patients and other health colleagues:

"[Role of health visitor] Mostly in [this town] at the moment it's the under fives, families with children under five that we visit when they've had their new babies and through until they've gone to school. A lot of the work is with the smaller end, the baby end of that in that that is where problems most often arise with the stress and coping with the new baby and the situation, but I know in my caseload there's a lot of child protection and a lot of work with families because of the problems of deprivation so I tend to see children perhaps more often in the older going up to school age range than most health visitors do. With the health problems, with the parenting skills, with the parents a lack of ... a lot of the parents have come out of a care situation. I'm also 'look after yourself' trained so I do take an interest in the adult end and would like to see more visiting with elderly or cardiac rehab patients or, y'know I would like to do a bit more variation but at the moment we're tied into families really with children under five." (Ms Lacey)

"As a practice nurse? A fairly multifaceted role, there's open access to me if anyone wants to see me anytime then my working hours there's no appointment system so they're free to visit or to call. The role involves healthcare, health promotion, general screening, diabetic screening, you do get involved with the families over a period of time because being a [small] practice we get to know our families." (Ms Naylor)

Both of these extracts identify the centrality of the family to the roles and responsibilities of non-medical health professionals. Both Ms Naylor and Ms Lacey also identify shifts towards health promotion and prevention of illness as central to their professional roles. The location of the responsibilities of both these professional groups have inherent within them the potential to address issues of domestic violence in relation to general family healthcare. However, while a theoretical shift has taken place to incorporate the concepts of health promotion and prevention, the role of the health visitor is still very much concerned on a practical level with issues of child welfare and child protection. The issue of age in relation to definitions of domestic violence was examined earlier. Both of these extracts illustrate how the differentiation between issues of child protection and domestic violence impacts on the ability of non-medical health professions to fulfil the potential of their professional responsibilities to a range of patient groups.

This chapter has examined the views of stage two participants in relation to general medical and non-medical roles and responsibilities, as well as knowledge relating to definitions of domestic violence. That these views do not exist within medical discourse in isolation has been evident throughout this discussion. The following chapter takes this issue further, by examining the explanations which healthcare professionals offer as to the causes of domestic violence.

Notes

[1] While a small number of healthcare professionals acknowledged having treated gay men for domestic violence-related injuries, none of the interviewees acknowledged treating lesbian women for such injuries.

[2] Area Child Protection Committee's (ACPCs) are inter-agency forums which emerged in order to improve the collaboration between professionals in relation to child protection issues. Derbyshire ACPC utilised this forum to address the issue of domestic violence and its impact on children at an ACPC-sponsored conference which took place on 20 April 1998.

[3] The fact that domestic violence has historically been referred to as a 'private' issue emanates from the distinction between the 'public' and 'private' spheres of social inclusion (Wollstonecraft, 1929; Mill, 1929) as legitimised within Liberal political thought. This distinction is responsible for excluding women from social participation and has also masked the reality that women are more likely to experience violence and abuse from men known to them than from strangers (Stanko, 1988). This distinction between the public/private spheres of social citizenship is important in relation to the occurrence of domestic violence, as it demonstrates the historical ways in which power and social control function in relation to individuals, the family and the state. Domestic violence was perceived as a private matter which was hidden from the public gaze and not therefore an area in which the state had a right to intervene.

[4] For a more detailed theoretical discussion about the medical hierarchy and gendered power within it, professionalisation, medicalisation and the emergence of the medical profession, see Williamson (1999).

SEVEN

Explanations of causes

As has already been suggested, the position of domestic violence within medical practice cannot be isolated from the social, cultural and legal discourses which shape how domestic violence is constructed as an individual and social phenomenon. Both groups of participants discussed within various contexts what they considered to be the causes of domestic violence. These responses include blaming or questioning the role of 'the victim' within the domestically violent situation, the personality traits of both the 'victim' and 'perpetrator', biological and hormonal explanations, cycle of abuse theories, individual characteristics of the perpetrator, environmental factors, social, economic, and cultural explanations and, finally, patriarchal analyses of domestic violence.

This chapter will examine the perceptions of the stage two participants in relation to the causes of domestic violence. The participants from stage one of the research did contribute to this discussion within their own interviews; however, this is not included in the text. Where differences and/or similarities exist between the two groups they will be examined. In the following discussion, the responses of the participating healthcare professionals will be contextualised with data which emerged from the domestic violence and health questionnaire sample, from which this in-depth sample originated[1].

Victim blaming and cycle of abuse theories

The following quotations focus on interview extracts which implicate 'the victim' in the cause of domestic violence. While focusing on the 'victim' of a legally defined crime may appear questionable, the actions of women who experience domestic violence have already appeared as significant in previous discussions. In Chapter Two, for example, 'victim' blaming was found by research conducted by Kurz (1987), in relation to the response of health practitioners to domestic violence. It was clear from the research on which this book is based that the participating women from stage one had internalised such theories and were aware of their impact.

> "I find it frustrating when some people choose, and again I'm stereotyping here, y'know you see some ... I don't know if it happens with men, but some women that seem to choose the same partner again, the same type of partner again and that's frustrating and when they go back that is just horrendous and that is going to add and clinically, like I've been round this circle before sort of thing, it's going to end up [in] violence or the death of somebody, or just a very unhappy situation." (Dr Jabber)

In the above extract Dr Jabber, while focusing on the motivations of the 'victim' of domestic violence, also suggests that women are somehow responsible for domestic violence through the life choices which they make. The cyclical relationship Dr Jabber describes suggests that not only do women fail to leave violent relationships, but when they do they continue to choose similar intimate partners again.

> "Some people fall into undesirable relationships and there are women who have multiple partners and they seem more at risk of violence because they tend to be unstable and violent types. I certainly see a number of those where you see that the situation is going to deteriorate anyway because the partners often has a ... violence already. We have had a number of those yet they still seem to fall in to relationships. They are often pregnant and intend to be pregnant." (Dr Fagan)

Dr Fagan's comments above are similar to those expressed by Dr Jabber in that he implicates women in 'choosing' violent partners. Both these extracts question the role that women play as 'victims' of domestic violence, whether that is to 'choose' violent and abusive partners or to perpetuate abusive relationships through their own behaviour. This type of 'victim blaming' is common, not only to domestic violence, but also to other gendered crimes and experiences (Schur, 1984; Lloyd, 1995). The ways in which the healthcare professionals above refer to the role 'victims' play in the causes of abuse and violence supports the literature from North America which documents how many women presenting with domestic violence-related injuries are ascribed stigmatising personality qualities which preclude their ability to receive support and information beyond basic clinical treatment (Kurz, 1987). Reliance on social stereotypes of women who experience domestic violence also questions the possibility of medicalising domestic violence in a context which does not also incorporate cultural myths about women:

"I know with some of the families that I visit, it always makes me surprised, I always think I know, 'Oh yeah, she's come from a care situation, it's happened, and then they don't have the parenting skills and then the level at which they operate, the silly little things that I take for granted that they don't know about that they haven't experienced and then that makes you stop and think that they haven't got the same set of rules that we have to play by, have they almost?" (Ms Lacey)

"I don't know … y'know there's a sort of, perhaps they've been abused themselves as youngsters, perhaps they see violence as a form of attention, they need attention, human contact and that's the only contact they understand and know, and therefore they sort of seek that type of behaviour in somebody again…." (Dr Jabber)

Both of the extracts above refer to the abusive histories of women as explaining the occurrence of domestic violence. These examples illustrate both 'victim blaming' and cycle of abuse theories in conjunction with one another. Ms Lacey also differentiates between women who experience domestic violence and herself by implying that 'they don't live their lives by the same rules'. Ms Lacey is therefore differentiating between herself and 'other' women, who experience domestic violence. This was suggested earlier, in Chapter Four, as one reason why some female nurses may respond negatively to women experiencing domestic violence.

Focusing on the ideologies present in theories which describe 'dysfunctional families' is something which was prevalent in the interviews of women who had experienced domestic violence and of healthcare professionals. Studies which have examined the significance of histories of violence and abuse, whether that has been to experience child abuse or witness domestic violence between adults, are inconsistent in their findings, which range from 24% (Hastings and Hamberger, 1988) to 81.1% (Roy, 1977) of violent men admitting experiencing domestic violence as a child. The effects of domestic violence on children who witness it is beyond the scope of this study[2]; however, without more consistent and thorough evidence, cycle of abuse theories cannot be utilised as an adequate explanation for the occurrence of domestic violence, as they do not explain why men who also experience domestic violence as children do not go on to abuse their own partners. The extracts above do suggest, however, that theories which purport to explain domestic violence through individualised concepts of 'victim blaming' and 'cycles of abuse' (Pizzey, 1974; Gayford, 1975a, 1975b; Pizzey and Shapiro, 1982) are firmly located within a domestic violence discourse which informs how women who experience domestic violence are perceived.

The ways in which social and cultural ideologies operate to control women and legitimate the ways in which individual men control women through violence and abuse, explains not only the existence of domestic violence but the wider social and political control of women. Focusing on the behaviour of 'victims' of violence enables healthcare professionals to legitimate cycle of abuse, and dysfunctional family theories which preclude the consideration of wider political and social explanations for the occurrence of violence. Women who experience domestic violence also appropriate these individualised theories as reasons for remaining with a violent partner, and in so doing perpetuate the idea that it is they who are deviant for staying. In retrospect, however, some women who experience domestic violence, and the majority of women who participated in this research, utilise sociopolitical theories to explain their abusive partners violent behaviour once they themselves have left such a relationship. Such explanations were absent in the healthcare professionals' interviews, where there was no discussion about social or political differentiations of power between men and women.

Environmental factors

The differentiation between the responses of both participant groups continued in relation to environmental and social causes of domestic violence. Some healthcare professionals suggested that alcohol, stress, money and socioeconomic position were significant contributing factors in the occurrence of domestic violence.

> "... but the violence angle that comes undoubtedly if you mix with certain company and if you behave in certain ways you are going to be far more at risk." (Dr Fagan)

Dr Fagan is differentiating between those people more likely to experience abuse and those who are not by focusing on the life-styles of his patients. He is also again implicating the 'victim' of abuse by assuming that she chooses to mix with certain people:

> "I know that it happens across social class and I know that it happens but I suppose with the area that I work in it doesn't feel like something

that can be taken out of context as the poverty and deprivation that are there because it feels like it's much worse if this man's totally in control of what income you've got if you've got no job that you could go to or no car that you can whiz out and get away, if you're tied to that man and the income comes from him and you're just on income support, that must weigh down much more heavily I think, if you're having to struggle for survival as well as cope with violence and that sort of thing." (Ms Lacey)

"They're often not necessarily the most articulate anyway, that can often be the case if we take it as an overall thing, no you can't say domestic violence only effects social class 4 and 5, it happens in 1-5 but perhaps it happens more in 4 and 5 doesn't it?" (Ms Naylor)

Ms Lacey's and Ms Naylor's comments are problematic as they are both aware that statistically social class is not a significant explanation for the occurrence of domestic violence (Dobash and Dobash, 1992; Mama, 1996). Despite this knowledge, they still find it difficult to dismiss this explanation, which identifies domestic violence as a problem for specific communities. Ms Lacey does, however, identify a number of problems which may be exacerbated within a domestically violent situation as a result of socioeconomic status[3].

"I think that there is a lot more violence out there that people actually accept. They don't actually want it dealing with and that is preventing us dealing with it more than anything else – the general public's perception of it should be an acceptable relationship will lead to areas within the practice where violence is perfectly acceptable to groups of people. Yet these are generally socioeconomic groups four and five, or six if there were one. We do have some very deprived areas and in those areas violence is more acceptable, particularly ex-miners, who have a very odd culture with regards to violence." (Dr Fagan)

The extract above is particularly interesting as Dr Fagan identifies not only social class as an explanation for domestic violence but the type of community where he perceives violence to be more acceptable. First, Dr Fagan's reference to a local mining community is interesting, because it could represent a belief that violence is related to the male/masculine culture of such industries. The acknowledgement of the impact of masculine identities within such industries would also therefore demonstrate an awareness of the gendered nature of violence and abuse. However, Dr Fagan is utilising this example to highlight areas of deprivation and unemployment within his surgery's catchment area and not to highlight the power relations inherent within the acquisition of gendered identities. Second, while it has been demonstrated earlier (in Chapter Four) that some women do not want 'help' from healthcare professionals, this is not the same as accepting domestic violence, as is implied in Dr Fagan's assertion. As has already been discussed, women who experience domestic violence negotiate and survive such relationships in a number of ways. Assuming that a reluctance to accept professional intervention represents an acceptance of such violence is to understate the resourcefulness of women who experience domestic violence as an everyday reality.

To summarise the other environmental factors which emerged within the second stage interviews, Ms Naylor, Ms Lacey and Dr Jabber all mentioned alcohol as a precipitating factor in the occurrence of domestic violence. Finally, both Dr Jabber and Dr Aaron referred to individual personality traits such as 'short fuses' as precipitating domestic violence incidents. While these explanations may explain the dynamics of domestic violence in specific individual cases, they do not offer us explanations which adequately explain the cause of domestic violence. The way in which individualised explanations for the occurrence of domestic violence are utilised can best be illustrated through research which has focused on the explanations men who beat their partners have given for their violent behaviour. Such research (Eiskovits and Edleson, 1989; Ptacek, 1988; Edleson and Tolman, 1992; The B Team, 1994; Mullender, 2000b) identifies the ways in which men use explanations for their violence which focus predominantly on the behaviour of the 'victim' or external factors, such as alcohol or drug abuse, rather than their own violent behaviour. This body of research also implicates the actions of professionals, in that other factors, such as the psychopathology of the perpetrator, are often utilised as explanations for the occurrence of domestic violence. The fact that such explanations are socially sanctioned, through both the criminal justice system and media representation of domestic violence, culminates in men utilising such explanations to justify and/or explain their violent behaviour. The researchers, identified above, who have examined in more detail the motivations of domestic violence perpetrators suggest that the explanations offered are often contradictory.

Despite the variety of theoretical perspectives that inform these works, all assume that the batterer loses control over his behaviour. This notion – that the batterer's will is somehow overpowered, that his violence lies outside of the realm of choice, that battering occurs during brief irrational episodes – constructs a contemporary profile of the batterer as one who is not necessarily sick, but who is rather just temporarily insane. Seen from this perspective, the batterer is not abnormal enough to be considered a psychopath and not responsible enough to be considered a criminal. But this notion of loss of control is substantially contradicted by the batterers' own testimony. While the men claim that their violence is beyond rational control, they simultaneously acknowledge that the violence is deliberate and warranted. (Ptacek, 1988, p 153)

This contradiction, evident within many perpetrators' testimonies, severely undermines the adequacy of individualistic explanations of the cause of domestic violence. This would include theories which focus on cycle of abuse and/or concepts of dysfunctional families. As with all of these explanations, it is important to consider the wider social and political framework within which domestic violence occurs. This includes acknowledging the historical and cultural acceptance of violence against women on a global scale. That such theories were relatively common in the interviews with stage two participants suggests that much more work needs to be conducted in challenging social myths and stereotypes about domestic violence, in the context of general basic awareness training.

Biological explanations

As well as the social and individualised theories and explanations offered by the participating healthcare professionals, one general practitioner also identified biological factors which he considered contributed to the causes of domestic violence.

"Well I think that you have to assess what the overriding need [is]. Do they need something to do with their depression? Do they need something to deal with their physical problems? Do they need something – in some cases hormone replacement therapy because it is actually menopausal symptoms which are provoking the whole situation? Once you settle those down and they then feel more comfortable then their relationship improves with their husband and the frustration and violence disappears." (Dr Fagan)

The biological explanation offered by Dr Fagan above suggests that domestic violence is related to the menopausal symptoms of women. If this were so, domestic violence would be limited to the experiences of women of a specific age and this is not the case (Mercy and Saltzman, 1989). Dr Fagan is explaining domestic violence through a biomedical model of healthcare which has medicalised women's very basic biological functions[4]. This biological explanation negates the possibility of incorporating a social or political explanation for the occurrence of domestic violence and places the responsibility of violence and abuse within a gendered biologically deterministic framework.

> "Quite often they present with a seemingly trivial condition and then go on to talk about what is worrying them. How they feel threatened or how they have been threatened. With women it is quite often that they will not give in to sexual demands and they are attacked as a consequence. That seems to be fairly frequent. It is more frequent that women get to forty and beyond and their sex drive seems to disappear and their partner's has not. I would say that I see more people suffer domestic violence mid-life than I do early on or late on." (Dr Fagan)

Dr Fagan's assumption that women are not sexually active beyond the age of 40 is both problematic and medically incorrect (Hite, 1977; Phillips and Rakusen, 1989). Both of these assertions are problematic because they imply that it is the hormonal differences between men and women which need to be addressed, through the manipulation of women's biology, to accommodate the biological drives and needs of men (Crawford, 1977; Candib, 1994). Biological theories do not, therefore, offer us adequate explanations and/or cures for domestic violence, but do highlight the problematic location of women within medical discourse.

The statistical prevalence of various explanations

The previous sections of this chapter have examined the responses which were given by the second stage participants as to the causes of domestic violence. Both participant groups identified similar explanations, including cycle of abuse theories and concepts of the 'dysfunctional family'. Sociocultural and environmental explanations were also proffered by both participant groups; however, the women from stage one also contextualised their responses in relation to sociopolitical explanations which incorporated a gendered analysis of domestic violence. Unfortunately, within the interviews with healthcare professionals, this type of consideration was lacking, and many healthcare professionals introduced explanations which focused on the 'victim' in order to construct a concept of conflicting families where the adults involved were ascribed equal responsibility for the occurrence of violence.

The responses of the participating healthcare professionals can also be viewed in the context of the results of the larger domestic violence and health questionnaire from which this stage two sample of healthcare professionals came (Abbott and Williamson, 1999). Respondents to this questionnaire were asked to consider a number of explanations and causes of domestic violence and to identify which they believed to be most common.

Box 8, by differentiating between the physical, sexual and mental elements of domestic violence, also enables us to examine how responsibility is differentiated by healthcare professionals in relation to the various manifestations of control within a domestically violent relationship. In relation to reasons which "underlie men physically assaulting their female partners", the most common explanation was relationship problems (24.7%), followed by male partner's psychological state (19.4%), and male partner's behaviour (17.6%). In relation to sexual assault, healthcare professionals identify the male partner's psychological state (24.4%), relationship problems (25.4%) and male partner's behaviour (19.9%) as the most common causes. The same three causes are prevalent in responses identifying the most common reason underlying men's mental cruelty, with male partner's psychological state (29.3%), relationship problems (24.4%) and male partner's behaviour (19.3%) the three most common responses. While the prevalence of the same responses within all three categories is interesting, the subtle differences within each is informative specifically in relation to explanations which directly attribute blame and cause to the female partner. In particular, 1% of respondents considered the most common cause of mental assault within a domestically violent relationship to be attributable to female psychology. This indicates that the biologically deterministic responses of Dr Fagan above need to be taken seriously. Also of relevance are responses which suggest the most common cause of domestic violence to be the female partner's behaviour and psychological state. This type of explanation can be observed in the interview extracts included above,

Box 8: Explanations as to the most common underlying cause of physical assault, sexual assault and mental cruelty within domestic violence (%)

Explanations	Physical assault	Sexual assault	Mental cruelty
Male partner's behaviour	17.6	19.9	19.3
Female partner's behaviour	0.2	0.5	1.2
Male psychological state	19.4	24.4	29.3
Female psychological state	0.2	0.5	1.5
Mental illness in male partner	1.7	1.9	2.9
Mental illness in female partner	–	–	1.0
Domestic circumstances	4.1	0.5	1.0
Social circumstances	12.5	1.9	5.9
Relationship problems	24.7	24.4	24.4
Subcultural norms	1.5	1.0	1.7
Situational response	3.2	3.6	2.9
Male socialisation	5.4	8.9	6.1
Male biology	0.2	5.5	0.2
Female biology	–	–	–
Other	9.2	6.2	3.4

which identify 'victim blaming' as an adequate explanation of domestic violence. The prevalence of relationship problems as an explanation within all three of the categories is congruent with the responses of the stage two participants in this study. The concept of relationship problems can be located in theories which identify dysfunctional family dynamics as responsible for the occurrence of domestic violence at the expense of focusing on the behaviour of the male perpetrator of such crimes.

Perceptions of domestic violence patients

It has been demonstrated throughout this and previous chapters that the healthcare professionals who participated in this research frequently implicated the behaviour of women presenting with domestic violence-related injuries in their explanations of the causes of domestic violence. This manifested itself through blaming women and the 'victims' of domestic violence, as well as advocating theories which centred around the problem of 'dysfunctional' families rather than focusing on the behaviour of the perpetrator of violence and abuse. Within the interviews conducted with healthcare professionals, I deliberately requested that they try to empathise with women who experience domestic violence, and try to explain how they might be feeling about both the abuse they experienced and the help-seeking process they were engaged in. The following extracts generally came in response to this question, although some of the quotations came from more general discussions within the interview process:

> "I hate to say it but it seems to be the same people over and over again, they're so accepting and just seem to go back for more which I never understand." (Dr Padden)

Dr Padden clearly finds the fact that women continue to experience domestic violence frustrating. The result of this frustration is that he finds it difficult to comprehend why women who experience domestic violence return to a violent relationship. The problem of asking this rather than other pertinent questions has already been raised in this text. Also, the impact of domestic violence on both the physical and non-physical well-being of women has also been addressed in the context of the wider experience of domestic violence. It is a reality that women who experience domestic violence frequently return to their abusers. McWilliams and McKiernan (1993) found that the majority of women in their study had left and returned to an abusive partner between two and six times. There are, however, a number of reasons for this. First, although women want the violence to end, this is not the same as wanting the relationship itself to end. Often after an abusive incident the perpetrator will demonstrate great remorse, which a woman who experiences domestic violence will want to believe is genuine. Second, women often have nowhere to go, which makes leaving a very practical problem. This is obviously compounded when children are involved. Third, if the abuser and society generally do not challenge the violence, it is very easy for a woman to understate the impact and danger of an abusive situation. These factors should also be considered within an historical context where domestic violence was not illegal, a fact which clearly influences the cultural discourses through which we understand domestic violence in contemporary society. Considering the fact that women remain within domestically violent relationships for a wide range of reasons, Dr Padden's frustrations, illustrated in the extract above, must make it very difficult for him to interact with the majority of domestic violence-related patients, many of whom will have returned to an abusive partner at some point. As was addressed in Chapter Four, the participating women from stage one were only too aware that professionals were frustrated by their returning to an abusive situation.

This perception of domestic violence-related patients is therefore understood and acknowledged by both participant groups. As such, it is a frustration which needs to be addressed by healthcare professionals through more transparent communications with their patients:

> "When someone comes in and brings their partner I find that sort of blame shifting to some extent because I think there's two sides to all these stories, you've got to get both partners apart at some time to get to the truth." (Dr Padden)

This extract from the interview with Dr Padden is interesting because it demonstrates how Dr Padden perceives domestic violence to be a phenomenon caused by the actions and behaviour of both parties. While Dr Padden may perceive this stance to demonstrate his own professional neutrality, women who experience domestic violence consider such a stance to be negative (Herman, 1992a) and therefore threatening.

> It is very tempting to take the side of the perpetrator. All the perpetrator asks is that the bystander do nothing.... The victim, on the contrary, asks the bystander to share the burden of pain. The victim demands action, engagement and remembering. (Herman, 1992a, pp 7–8)

Considering the argument made in the quotation above, the motivation behind Dr Padden's wish to see both sides of the patient's story can be called into question. The neutrality he aspires to is impossible within a situation where power is already unevenly distributed between those involved.

Understanding the impact of domestic violence

Dr Habberley, Ms Naylor, and Dr Jabber all identified emotions such as guilt, shame, depression, anxiety, fear, resentment, bitterness, and anger as important emotions which will be experienced by women experiencing domestic violence. They also acknowledged the effects that these emotions have on a woman's subjective experience through loss of self-esteem and confidence and also the impact of silencing. Asking healthcare professionals to discuss how they perceive women who present with domestic violence-related injuries, and what they think about such patients, was important in order to identify first, whether the participating women's perceptions of the medical interaction were valid and second, to identify the effects of the health interaction/ professional, on the presenting women's sense of self. The following extracts are extremely positive, as they identify instances where healthcare professionals have seriously considered the wider implications of domestic violence on the presenting 'victim', and also the impact of their own professional role on that experience:

"That's definitely true, my point is about utilisation of us as a resource and how certain things take up our time that might be inappropriately managed, or managed elsewhere, but your point about how difficult it is to disclose is very well made and that's absolutely right and I'm sure its very hard to make that first step to tell somebody that you're in a threatening situation and it must be hard because if it wasn't, people would be getting out, they wouldn't need to tell because if it was an easy thing to do they'd be making alternative choices, so we can extrapolate from that that it's a hard situation to be in and part of our job is to be, to make patients aware that we trust their confidentiality, we respect them as individuals and that we will try and help but only to the limits of what they want and if that point could get across then people might be less fearful of disclosing to us." (Dr Gabb)

"Obviously they would like it to stop so that they are concerned about the future, concerned about breaking up even if it is a violent relationship, they are concerned about breaking up a relationship and where they are going to live. Where the children are going to be and so on. I think that that is about it. Oh yes they might be concerned about my own attitude. Is he going to listen to me, or you know, so they often put out a few opening gambits to see how receptive to what they have come about really." (Dr Iannelli)

Both of these extracts demonstrate how not all the healthcare professionals who participated in this study relied on cultural myths to explain domestic violence. Both Dr Gabb and Dr Iannelli are aware of the effects domestic violence has on those who experience it, and locate their professional practice in relation to those feelings and experiences. Dr Gabb, in particular, extends this professional responsibility within a wider inter-agency context (this will be discussed in Chapter Twelve) which is extremely positive. Also in the above extract from Dr Gabb, we can observe how she considers how difficult it is to disclose information about domestic violence, and that it is the social context of domestic violence which results in women returning to health practitioners.

In relation to the frustrations which are evident in all of the interview extracts in this chapter, healthcare professionals who do not consider the existence of domestic violence within a wider social context find such health interactions frustrating. The irony, however, is that with few real choices, women who experience domestic violence will continue to present to a range of professionals for help and advice. The continuation of such presentations, without reflexive consideration by the health professional as to why, results in an escalation of professional frustration which could be avoided. It is interesting that while only a small number of the participating healthcare professionals considered the impact of the health interaction on the presenting patient, the majority of stage one participants acknowledged the frustrations which dealing with domestic violence-related injuries cause for health professionals. This discrepancy highlights how both participant groups internalise the culturally sanctioned explanations and causes discussed above, and incorporate them in their interactions with each other. The following chapters examine health professionals' views of this interaction, and of domestic violence-related injuries generally.

Notes

[1] Also see Abbott and Williamson (1999) for a more detailed analysis of this data.

[2] Those participating women who had children talked at length in their interviews about the role of their children in the decisions they themselves made and the impact of domestic violence on their children, both during childhood and as adults.

[3] While environmental factors may not offer an adequate explanation for the cause of domestic violence, such factors clearly influence the help-seeking alternatives available to women who experience domestic violence.

[4] For a discussion relating to the medicalisation of women, see Riessman (1983), Warshaw (1992) and Candib (1994).

EIGHT

Physical versus non-physical injuries

Part One identified the experiences of the stage one participants in relation to their clinical interactions with healthcare professionals. A number of issues were acknowledged, including the extent of physical and non-physical injuries which the participating women ascribed to the domestic violence they were experiencing. This chapter is intended to address those concerns from the perceptions of the stage two participants. As such, it addresses the identification and diagnosis of physical and non-physical injuries within a number of contexts.

Identifying physical injuries

Before looking at the way in which the participating healthcare professionals identified physical domestic violence-related injuries, it should be acknowledged that all of the participating general practitioners and health visitors had experience of dealing with domestic violence-related injuries in their clinical practice. Within the wider sample of respondents to the domestic violence and health questionnaire (Abbott and Williamson, 1999), 15.5% of respondents believed they saw women who had *physical injuries* as a result of assault by their male partner at least once a month, 76% occasionally, and 8.5% believed they never treated women who had physical injuries as a result of domestic violence. Clearly, therefore, most healthcare professionals will, at least occasionally, treat women who have physical injuries caused by domestic violence. Considering this revelation, I asked all of the healthcare professionals what types of injuries they had been presented with and/or what types of injuries would make them suspect that domestic violence was a possible cause of injury. They identified similar injuries and were competent at identifying non-accidental injuries:

> "Patients would usually disclose but if not would look for physical injuries, separate injuries in various locations. Look initially for facial injuries, ie black eyes, pressure marks to upper arms, blows to the head, would apply the same rules as to child protection." (Dr Aaron)

"Well, obviously unexplained injuries that I came across in the examination. If she said that she had come in with a cough and I listened to her chest and then I found that she had a lot of bruises of various ages then that would suggest some sort of violence, domestic violence." (Dr Iannelli)

"... there may be the obvious signs of physical abuse, the bruise, black eye, 'oh, I did that bumping into the door' or something like that and clearly it's inconsistent what they're actually saying." (Dr Jabber)

"... a very difficult situation working out what kind of injuries are to look out for like fingertip bruising and that kind of thing." (Dr Eagland)

The participating healthcare professionals were able to identify specific types of injuries including fingertip bruising, bruising to the wrists, bruising to the eyes, broken ribs, inappropriate scratching, and bruising generally as possible indicators that domestic violence was the cause of an injury. The implications of whether or not they act on this information will be discussed further in Chapter Nine; however, healthcare professionals are clearly competent at identifying when domestic violence is a likely cause of a physical injury which they might be presented with.

While one practice nurse identified that she may come across incidents of sexual abuse during the administering of cervical smear tests, none of the general practitioners identified specific health services where domestic violence was presented more often than others. This is unfortunate, as we know from statistical evidence (Webster et al, 1994; Chez, 1994; Norton et al, 1995) that domestic violence is more likely to occur when a women is or becomes pregnant. Indeed, three of the participating women from stage one, Carol, Iris and Helena, had experienced physical domestic violence during pregnancy. One midwife[1] was interviewed in the second stage and, although she was conscious that domestic violence was a health issue did not perceive this to be specifically related to prenatal care. She also felt that, due to the limited time that midwives spend with individual women, she would not necessarily be in the best position to identify domestic violence or act upon it. This again raises the issue of continuity of care. Fortunately, the Royal College of Obstetrics and Gynaecology has published one of the first comprehensive British texts examining domestic violence and health (Friend et al, 1998). This suggests that there are British health professionals within prenatal and gynaecological services who do recognise the importance of domestic violence during pregnancy, in relation to the health of both the mother and fetus. As mentioned in Chapter Three, the impact of domestic violence on the health of pregnant women goes beyond pregnancy itself and impacts on a whole range of reproductive and sexual choices. This suggests that all health professionals working in services related to reproductive and sexual services need to be aware of the impact of domestic violence on their patients.

Although this text is concerned with the treatment offered and received by women who experience domestic violence, there are obviously adverse health implications for the misdiagnosis of injuries and their long-term effects more generally.

"Sometimes you see people that come in with a bandage around the wrist. I am always interested why they have got a bandage around the wrist because it might not only be associated with violence but often the first signs of neurological complaints, can be frequent burning, accidental burns. People just misjudge things, so we want to know how people have done what they seem to be trivial injuries in places that you would not expect them. Anybody can cut a finger but the wrist is quite an unusual place to injure unless you are particularly clumsy or you have been deliberately handled in that area. A history of a fall, might be a good history of a fall and would have no reason to think that it is nothing other than that. It is when the injury does not match the story that they give that I would begin to ask more detailed questions about how that they got it." (Dr Fagan)

The extract from the interview with Dr Fagan above suggests that identifying the cause of an injury to the wrist is important, as it could be an indication of other serious and long-term health problems. It is likely, therefore, that identifying domestic violence as the cause of an injury assists in eliminating other possibilities as well as addressing injuries before they develop into long-term health problems. The long-term health effects of domestic violence as experienced by the participating women from stage one were examined in Chapter Three. As the extract above demonstrates, intervention at an early stage can eliminate alternative diagnoses and ensure that appropriate treatment is offered for a domestic violence-related injury.

Psychosomatic complaints

The women who constituted the first stage research participants identified numerous psychosomatic complaints including eating disorders, weight loss, anxiety, depression, sleeping disorders, panic attacks, neurotic behaviour and general feelings of illness as physical symptoms which they attributed to domestic violence. While healthcare professionals were competent at identifying domestic violence from physical injuries, I was particularly interested in whether they would take seriously the association between psychosomatic injuries and domestic violence. In the domestic violence and health questionnaire (Abbott and Williamson, 1999), respondents were asked to identify the frequency with which they treated women who presented with *mental health problems* as a result of harassment/violence/cruelty by their male partner. In response, 14.8% stated at least once a month, 72.2% occasionally, and 8.8% never. Comparing these responses to those highlighted above, in relation to the frequency with which healthcare professionals believed they treated physical injuries, the questionnaire sample considered they treated mental health-related injuries less frequently than physical injuries. This is an interesting finding as it does not correspond to the experiences of the stage one participants of this research. Non-physical injuries were more prominent in the stage one women's accounts of their experiences of domestic violence and health, and more women had had contact with mental health services than with, for example, accident and emergency departments:

> "Yes, well I would certainly try and [determine] a cause if someone was coming in with excessive anxiety or insomnia or depression. Any of those of the neurosis. You know domestic violence could be a cause of that. I would just ask generally is there anything at home that is upsetting you, or anything at work and tackle it that way." (Dr Iannelli)

> "... more their attitude as they come in, these people are often presenting depression or hidden depression, vague abdominal pains, headaches which we do the standard investigations and rule out the clinical pathology but at the end of the day it's often a depressive cause and then you try and get to the root of the problem, have you got problems at work, have you got problems at home and eventually you wheedle it out but quite often it takes multiple visits." (Dr Padden)

"Like if someone's tearful when they come to see you and if they're depressed sometimes it will just be a casual remark that's enough to open the flood-gates. It's difficult to know if it's just clinical depression or something specific." (Ms Naylor)

"Sometimes, I suppose it's not always the obvious things sometimes you pick up that they're depressed or whatever." (Ms Lacey)

Many of the healthcare professionals offered psychosomatic complaints such as anxiety and depression as indicators of domestic violence in their initial response to questions relating to physical injuries. Those who did not were willing to accept that very often they are presented with women who experience domestic violence and who do not present with a physical injury caused by such abuse. These women were referred to in one instance as 'weepy women', and the manner in which they disclosed, or not, was clearly a cause for concern, as healthcare professionals can often find it frustrating. Healthcare professionals are, however, competent in identifying non-physical injuries, which manifest themselves through psychosomatic complaints, as being caused in many instances by the presence of domestic violence. While this is an encouraging finding, the lack of knowledge about domestic violence results in an understanding of domestic violence symptoms within existing psychological theories. This can frequently result in the underestimation of the effects of domestic violence as the cause of psychological injury. Various theorists (Maris, 1971; Walker, 1979, 1991; Tuan, 1984; Herman, 1992a, 1992b; Saunders, 1994; Stark and Flitcraft, 1995, 1996) have examined the psychological impact of domestic violence on women. Much of this research has also examined psychological complaints such as depression, chronic suicidality, borderline, dependent, passive-aggressive, masochistic and multiple personality disorders (Walker, 1979, 1991; Herman, 1992b). These examples of psychological illnesses are identified within disease categorisations which can often be confused with elements of the complex post-traumatic stress disorder manifest in the behaviour of women experiencing domestic violence. The problems associated with the misdiagnosis of psychosomatic injuries in cases of domestic violence have been discussed already in this book; it is relevant, however, to reiterate these concerns here.

"Absolutely, lots to be honest [sigh] I mean I wouldn't like to put a figure on it ... as far as the physical violence is concerned I could probably say once every two or three months there's someone comes in with signs of physical violence. As far as sort of mental cruelty, violence, I probably see two or three cases a week of people coming in, 'I've had a bit of a row, a bit of a fall out, they've kicked me out again'." (Dr Padden,)

From the extract above the impact of non-physical injuries in terms of health provision is significant. Any health-specific definition of, or guidelines relating to, domestic violence must therefore identify, not only the physical health problems caused by domestic violence, but also the non-physical injuries, which manifest themselves through a wide variety of psychosomatic complaints.

Para-suicide

It was demonstrated in Chapters Six and Seven that healthcare professionals often assume a woman experiencing domestic violence should leave abusive relationships. Such opinions do not take into consideration the health impact, in terms of psychological injury, which women who present with domestic violence-related injuries are suffering. As the following extracts demonstrate, some healthcare professionals assume that the para-suicidal activities of women are not genuine, and they come to this conclusion by ignoring the underlying psychological processes which are impacted by a domestically violent situation.

While the number of stage one research participants who had experience of para-suicide may appear alarming (see Appendix 1, Table A1), and I was initially skeptical that this participant group's experiences were typical, statistics from North America identify domestic violence as a significant factor in the suicide and attempted suicide rates of women. This research varies in its design, but research comparing battered and non-battered female samples presenting to the medical profession has established that "one battered woman in six (17%) had attempted suicide and a significant proportion had done so multiple times" (Stark and Flitcraft, 1996, p 100). Other studies which focus on the experiences of women living in refuges (or their equivalent) have found that 35% to 40% have attempted suicide, a far higher figure than within the general female population (Gayford, 1975b; Walker, 1979). This literature focuses specifically on the issue of domestic violence; research which examines suicide more generally demonstrates that domestic violence is an important aetiological factor in that "80% of those who attempt suicide give marital or boyfriend or girlfriend conflicts as their reason" (Stark and Flitcraft, 1996, p 103).

> "I was also working as a ward sister in an area but we had a bed that was reserved for overdoses so from that angle I have a lot to do with female patients, because it was a female ward of patients. But the overdoses were often simple cries for help as much as the phenomenal violence that might be taking place later on, a lot of the youngsters were lots of sort of boyfriend problems and sometimes it's something that you can help them with because it is such a simple, fairly straightforward trigger factor that has caused them to take their overdose." (Ms Naylor)

The extract above demonstrates how 'relationship problems' are recognised by healthcare professionals as a 'trigger' to suicidal activity. Suicide and para-suicidal activity are important elements of the health response to domestic violence and the gendered power distinctions manifest in domestically violent relationships.

Despite the overwhelming experience of the stage one participants from this research, and also the statistical evidence which exists from other countries, the healthcare professionals who I interviewed were reluctant to move from the diagnosis of non-physical psychosomatic injuries relating to domestic violence to the acknowledgement that suicide and para-suicide were significant health issues in relation to domestic violence.

> "I do not think that I have seen anybody in 12 years who was attempting suicide because of domestic violence. I would not, I certainly do not see that as a main problem here. All the self-harm people that I see here are mentally ill. Two are just manipulative. They are not actually mentally ill, they are doing it for attention – and these are people in mid-life that just have an abnormal way of coping with things, but I do not see, no I have not seen any women attempting to get away from domestic violence situation by committing suicide." (Dr Fagan)

Dr Fagan's reluctance to make a connection between female suicide attempts and domestic violence was a common theme in the second stage interviews. Dr Fagan's comments are also disconcerting, as they do not take into account the need for women who experience domestic violence to be in control of their help-seeking activities. Such activities, if considered out of context, could be considered manipulative. As demonstrated earlier (Herman, 1992a), the behaviour of women who have experienced domestic violence, rather than being perceived as a stigmatising quality within the woman herself, should be considered as 'normal' responses to abuse within a violent context. Dr Fagan also considers this possibility only in terms of women attempting suicide to escape domestically violent situations. As demonstrated in Chapter Three, women's para-suicidal activity, while it may be rooted in domestic violence, is about the self-identity and subjective needs and experiences of the individual concerned, and not necessarily a direct way to leave an abusive partner.

While some healthcare professionals acknowledged there may be a problem with domestic violence and para-suicide, they were extremely reluctant to do so. The following extract demonstrates this reluctance, when a general practitioner told me minutes after denying the significance of my question that he in fact did have clinical experience of patients (male and female) who had attempted suicide in the context of a domestically violent situation:

> "I haven't actually had any women ... consistently sort of doing that. I've actually found women although they're upset and distressed we actually deal with it, they're usually more sort of anxious, depressed, clinical depression, want the support of an agency, they want to go through their feelings and acknowledge the fact that what they're feeling is normal, in a sense there's a bereavement process as well, there's a loss of esteem, there's guilt, there's a whole range of sort of feelings that they sort of go through. Interesting enough all of my patients who attempt suicide more than once will be men and they've been on sort of self-destruct mode for a variety of reasons. So, I can't think of a woman in surgery ... I'm sure there are but most of them present with all the other sort of mental health issues that perhaps heads it off before it gets that far? I don't know." (Dr Jabber)

> "... interestingly just as I said I haven't had any women try suicide, she did once just once though, but the whole, the both of them, he's tried it a couple of times, and I think she's tried it once." (Dr Jabber)

While acknowledging the contradiction above, it is interesting that Dr Jabber considers the response of healthcare professionals to be adequate. His belief that women will access help in a less traumatic context is not supported by the participating women's own testimonies, and raises questions about the adequacy of the medical response to domestic violence for those women who do not find support through other routes.

Not all of the participating healthcare professionals were uncomfortable with the connection between para-suicides and domestic violence. Ms Naylor, a practice nurse, and Dr Eagland, a female general practitioner, were both willing to acknowledge the impact of domestic violence within para-suicide cases. Dr Eagland also extends this acknowledgement to issues of self-harm more generally, which, as the extracts from the participating stage one women demonstrated, is an important connection to make.

> "I suppose sometimes they might tell me that they're frightened by what their partner's going to do ... sometimes they tell me that they live with a partner who's violent who has hit them or might hit them, [or] is just horrible. I would listen and take it into account in the treatment. I specifically ask people about self-harm, ask whether they're feeling suicidal thoughts." (Dr Eagland)

Dr Eagland's approach acknowledges the risk of para-suicide and self-harm in cases where domestic violence is an issue. This is 'good practice' and should be acknowledged as such. The following extract from Ms Naylor relates to her previous clinical experience and clearly validates the interpretations which the presenting women place on the healthcare interactions they have experienced, especially in relation to para-suicidal activity.

> "The first time that I actually met an overdose patient I think I'd been a student nurse for about eight weeks and I was on my first ward placement and I was sent on the afternoon to give this young girl, she'd be about 14,15, a suppository, now the relevance in relation to her overdose or anything else I couldn't reasonable comment on, it's totally irrelevant thing to do perhaps it's supposed to be some sort of punishment because she was using up a hospital bed, but I'm trying to put this into the equation of how things have evolved over say 20 years in relation to dealing with that so, and because I haven't got any knowledge and although I couldn't relate to her at all except that it was very difficult to give her these things because they kept flying all over the bed, but the general hospital approach or the healthcare approach was nothing like as sympathetic then as it is now. I think we have become a lot more aware about what we're

doing and at least trying to tune in and give appropriate sort of care." (Ms Naylor)

The example above is extreme, but locates historically the view of consistent female para-suicide patients. While such activity may not be tolerated now, 20 years later, it is not surprising considering its historical origins that the perception of (female) para-suicidal patients is one which stigmatises the patient. The practice identified by Ms Naylor above obviously influences the discourse around suicidal women's behaviour and informs the responses which women received in their interactions with healthcare professionals.

This chapter has introduced the responses of healthcare professionals to questions which emerged from interviews with women who had themselves experienced domestic violence. Much of the knowledge evident here comes from clinical practice and illustrates how practitioners have developed their responses to domestic violence, despite a lack of uniform policy and guidelines. Chapter Nine develops this clinical knowledge further, by examining how health practitioners approach the treatment of the domestic violence-related injuries identified here.

Notes

[1] In comparison to the number of other healthcare professionals, the number of midwives who were contacted and responded to the domestic violence and health questionnaire, from which the second stage research participants were recruited, was considerably less.

NINE

Treatment options

The stage one participants' experiences of treatment were examined in Chapter Four. This identified a number of treatments which they had been offered, and examined how they perceived such treatment in relation to their wider health interactions. This chapter will examine the treatment options which the participating healthcare professionals identified as central to their own clinical practice.

All of the stage two participants were asked prior to their participation in this qualitative study to answer questions on the domestic violence and health questionnaire in relation to how they treat domestic violence patients (Abbott and Williamson, 1999). The first of these questions asked what the respondents usually did in their professional capacity when dealing with women 'who had experienced cruelty or violence from a male partner'. From a number of given options, a small percentage (2.4%) believed they had 'no role' to play, 13.4% claimed they would treat the physical injury, 93.9% suggested they would provide information on available services, and 49.1% believed they should refer patients onto other agencies[1]. These responses were interesting, particularly when considered in relation to the subsequent questions relating to whether the respondents had adequate knowledge about services and local provision. Eight-six per cent of the respondents did not believe they had adequate knowledge of domestic violence. This is despite the fact that 93.9% suggested they would provide information on available services. Furthermore, 84.3% had never been involved in inter-agency work on domestic violence. The issue of inter-agency collaboration will be examined in Chapter Twelve; however, this statistic seriously undermines the ability of almost half of respondents (49.1%) to refer women to other agencies. In light of these responses, the qualitative data on which this book is based asked a series of questions designed to investigate the preferred treatment options, and perceptions of these alternatives by the stage two participants.

General responses

> "Sometimes of course there's physical treatment involved, attending to wounds, but not very often and then the third category are people who've been sent by the police or solicitors to get a record made and they just come in and say 'I'm alright but I just want you to write down that I've got these bruises or whatever, as a record', and out of all those categories it's the first one which is supportive counselling which I suppose I do the most of." (Dr Gabb)

The extract above differentiates between three different approaches which relate to the needs of the presenting patient. Dr Gabb identifies the need to address physical injuries, psychological well-being and the need to record domestic violence injuries for documentation purposes (documentation will be addressed in Chapter Ten). This type of multi-pronged approach towards the treatment of domestic violence injuries and the medical interaction between healthcare professionals was common among general practitioners' responses to this question. The following extract also illustrates the three most common responses from healthcare professionals.

> "My first priority was checking that the children were safe and OK. My second priority were the physical injuries and I suppose not counselling but in a very broad sense, but just talking to them seeing if I can be of any help in that situation.... Well I suppose normally if someone came in with an injury that looked as if it had been the result of violence, if someone comes in with a black eye or something then normally I try and find out how they got it. If they give a plausible explanation then if that's what they wanted me to believe then I'd probably leave it at that. If I thought there was more going on I might try and probe." (Dr Eagland)

The extract from Dr Eagland, like that from Dr Gabb, illustrates the tendency to address both physical and non-physical injuries through a broad-based counselling approach to interaction with women who have experienced domestic violence. Dr Eagland also identifies the discrepancies which arise when the patient does not disclose information about the cause of her particular injuries. This identifies the contradictions which exist in relation to domestic violence where, on purely medical grounds, the health professional is reluctant to investigate domestic violence where the presenting woman may be reluctant to disclose. This occurrence is not restricted to the experience of domestic violence. Issues of patient compliance, lay beliefs in relation to health, and the power inherent within the relationships between patients and professionals are fraught with difficulties (Salmon et al, 1994; Donahue and McGuire, 1995; Peters et al, 1998).

> "... you really need to tackle the set up at home, children, who is at home. What might have precipitated the attack, or attacks and maybe try to do something to prevent them in the future." (Dr Iannelli)

The above extract by Dr Iannelli is problematic; although it may appear to represent a proactive stance towards domestic violence it is possible to interpret the extract as locating responsibility for the violence on the 'victim'. This was demonstrated by Iris, who felt that her own general practitioner was assuming she could take responsibility for the violence she experienced and that she could avoid or prevent further attacks. The fallacy that there exists an adequate explanation for domestic violence, which can be identified in order to prevent it, has also been discussed throughout, and is an important consideration when making suggestions that women can prevent future attacks against them.

It is also interesting that in both the above extracts, Dr Eagland and Dr Iannelli mention the importance of children. While the need to protect children was evident in a number of stage two interviews, none of the healthcare professionals considered the 1989 Children's Act to be relevant in offering an impetus to safeguard the well-being of women experiencing domestic violence when they were the children's carer. This is unfortunate, as we know from research (Hendricks-Matthews, 1993; Straus and Smith, 1993; Zuckerman et al, 1995; Hester and Radford, 1996; Mullender et al, 2000) that the impact on children of witnessing domestic violence has long-term implications for their health and welfare. Healthcare professionals do not have legal responsibility for adults experiencing domestic violence (as they do for children experiencing abuse), yet acknowledging the parameters of the Children's Act, for example, in terms of moral, ethical and social responsibilities is an issue for professions which are attempting to change and reorganise their practice to fulfil the needs of patients in relation to a number of non-medicalised complaints.

Disclosure and communication

The most frequent response from the healthcare professionals who were interviewed was that they would listen to the presenting patient, offer a sympathetic ear, or counselling support. In response to questions examining the preferred treatment alternatives of the respondents in the domestic violence and health questionnaire (Abbott and Williamson, 1999), 33.2% stated they would advise a client/patient to receive counselling, and a further 36.1% believed they should counsel the woman themselves[2]. While the participating women generally perceived this type of support as positive (as addressed in Chapter Four), this approach was frequently combined with the assumption that it is the patient's responsibility to diagnose the origins of her injury. The problematic nature of this stance on disclosure is exacerbated when dealing with non-physical injuries. 74.7% of respondents to the domestic violence and health questionnaire stated that there were circumstances under which they would "directly ask a woman if she was experiencing physical, sexual and/or mental cruelty from her male partner". When asked to identify these circumstances, 35.6% stated they would ask if there was an unexplained injury, 13% if the patient was anxious or depressed, 4.8% if the patient had recurring attendance at the surgery, 0.4% if the patient was reliant on tranquillisers, 5.2% if she was evasive, 3.4% if there was evidence of relationship problems, and 0.2% if her male partner had alcohol or drug problems. A number of health professionals identify anxiety and depression as important, but none stated that they would ask about abuse as a matter of course. As the responses from the stage one participants demonstrated in Chapter Four, there were a number of occasions when the women were not asked about the cause of their injury, and felt their experiences were not therefore validated. Disclosure is therefore a very important issue which needs to be addressed by healthcare professionals, particularly in relation to screening and the identification of health needs within the general patient population.

> "If I suspected it [domestic violence], which is a big if to start with, I would be very disinclined to say 'Are you experiencing domestic violence?'. Firstly I don't think that's a very good question which begs yes or no, what I'd be more inclined to say is 'Is everything alright at home?', 'Is there anything else you want to tell me before you go?', 'You seem to have come several times in the last month, I'm not sure if I'm helping, is there anything else you want to tell me that might change what I'm doing?' If I get blank no's on the

day it's not to say I'll get blank no's the next time I see them, so all I have to do is indicate a willingness to listen and then leave it up to the patient. Sometimes if I know the patient well enough, I mean that's why it depends on the patient and your relationship and it's sometimes possible to say 'He's not beating you up is he?' and then they either break into floods of tears or they laugh it off, if they do the latter then that's either the end of it or they'll be in next time, 'Y'know what you were saying about ... well actually yes'. There are so many different ways." (Dr Gabb)

This extract acknowledges the difficulties which patients have in disclosing information about domestic violence. In relation to counselling, healthcare professionals need to be aware of a range of issues in order to understand the dynamics of domestic violence and assist the help-seeking processes of their patients. This includes acknowledging that women may be reluctant to disclose the origins of their domestic violence-related injuries.

Research from North America has examined approaches to the subject of domestic violence within health interactions, and has demonstrated that healthcare professionals need to ask direct and sensitive questions rather than indirect and vague ones. The findings of the research on which this text is based are similar to findings found in studies conducted in other countries (McIlwaine, 1989; Denham, 1995; Fishwick, 1995; Parsons et al, 1995). Healthcare professionals often feel uncomfortable asking patients about domestic violence, despite screening being an important part of their medical role and an important part of offering sympathetic advice (Tilden and Shepherd, 1987; Lazzaro and McFarlane, 1991; AMA, 1992; Hendricks-Matthews, 1993; Sheridan, 1993; Butler, 1995; Delahunta, 1995). It has been found that "although women do not willingly offer information about an abusive situation, they want to be asked about this intimate problem" (Drake, 1982, p 45). Communication between healthcare professionals and presenting domestic violence patients needs to be be improved. A good place to start is to question the reluctance of healthcare professionals to screen for domestic violence, despite the repeat presentation of injuries which results from such violence and the frustrations which that causes, not to mention the financial cost of such repeat presentations (Stanko et al, 1998). While barriers limit the responses a professional may offer a presenting patient, as the discussion in Chapter Seven acknowledged, healthcare professionals' previous experiences frequently result in frustrations which limit their clinical response prior to the medical interaction itself. Healthcare professionals are aware, therefore, of the difficulties facing women who experience domestic violence, but are reluctant to alter their patient interactions to counterbalance these difficulties (Schornstein, 1997). This issue can be located within debates around patient (consumer) compliance generally (Peters et al, 1998), and the power inherent within the medical encounter (Lupton, 1997). In relation to domestic violence, however, the appropriateness of healthcare professionals offering 'counselling' to patients needs to be addressed in relation to their reluctance to screen for domestic violence and assumptions about patient responsibility in relation to disclosure.

Dissemination of information and advice

Another element of the health interaction referred to by health professionals was the need to disseminate information and advice to patients. In the domestic violence and health questionnaire study (Abbott and Williamson, 1999), 93.9% of respondents believed they should inform women about available services. However, the amount of information and knowledge concerning local domestic violence service provision varied among the participant group. As already mentioned, 86% of respondents believed they did not have adequate knowledge of the services available to women who experience domestic violence. Healthcare professionals had more information about statutory services, such as the police and social services, than they did about voluntary services such as refuge provision, advice lines, and support groups (this will be examined in more detail in relation to inter-agency collaborations in Chapter Twelve).

> "I am there as a resource in a way of health information and I'm not there to judge the situation they're in or to explore necessarily ways to get out of it, because that's not always what they want. My job is to respond to help the patient figure out what is going on and is it what they want and deal with it in their way." (Dr Gabb)

Providing useful information to women who have experienced domestic violence requires specialist knowledge about specific services. It was not clear in interviews with the second stage participants that the majority of participants had such a knowledge base and, as the statistics above illustrate, the majority of respondents were not confident about the information they did possess.

"I don't think I've had enough knowledge or training to specifically offer advice or possible outcomes but I could point them in the direction of other services, possibly social services." (Ms Naylor)

Ms Naylor, a health visitor, identified that she believed she did not have enough specialised knowledge to deal with the issue of domestic violence. This is evident in her suggestion of accessing social services rather than other more specialised domestic violence services which exist locally. It was clear during the course of the stage two interviews that although general practitioners with less knowledge about domestic violence than Ms Naylor were happy to intervene and offer advice and broad-based counselling, Ms Naylor was not comfortable dealing with an issue which she had inadequate knowledge of. This raises a number of questions about the roles of the different participating professionals and the relationships between them. These issues will be addressed in Chapter Eleven.

Women/patient-centred treatments

Despite the problems discussed above, many of the healthcare professionals were sensitive about the needs of women presenting with domestic violence-related injuries, and advocated women-centred decisions about the treatment options available within the health interaction.

"Yes, probably more people of the counselling type who can you know, and you know I mean counselling in the proper sense in that they can help the woman to come to a decision about what she wants to do herself really. I don't think that pills are the answer. You can give prescriptions and antidepressants but they are not the real answer I don't think." (Dr Iannelli)

This extract from an interview with Dr Iannelli is extremely encouraging as it questions the use of drugs, and antidepressant drugs in particular, to treat women who experience domestic violence. Unfortunately, having moved away from the use of psychiatric drugs, Dr Iannelli's alternative is to advocate professional counselling, albeit to provide a patient-centred treatment plan. It appears, therefore, that it is extremely difficult for healthcare professionals to denounce the use of psychiatric alternatives, whether that be drugs or counselling, which too frequently offer a short-term solution to the problems presented by women patients, but which also abdicate responsibility for the patient away from the general practitioner. This effectively precludes the possibility of the health professional validating the presenting woman's experience by advocating a professional response. These issues are important, as the participating health professionals are advocating the dissemination of information and counselling, as medical responses, when the presenting women want their experiences validated within a social context.

> "First of all you've got to get them to admit that it's [domestic violence] part of the problem and that it is part of the hidden agenda that this might be going on and then once you've found out that that is a part of it, there are hundreds of ways of dealing with it but most of them will be directed to me by the patient and if all she wants to do is tell me about it then that's the end of it and I wouldn't involve anybody else. If what they need is in-depth counselling to come to terms with it then I would probably send her to [the community psychiatric nurse]. I don't tend very often to include anybody else. I know that there are resources available to me and that there are, for example, support groups and literature but I would be very much guided by how the patient sees the issue." (Dr Gabb)

The above extract is encouraging, as it advocates women-centred treatment and acknowledges the sensitive nature of domestic violence in terms of ongoing safety requirements. The following extract is less encouraging, as there is a difference in the perception of the presenting women. Rather than being supportive of patients, the following extract advocates 'doing nothing' unless instructed otherwise by the presenting patient.

> "I often don't know what they come for. Because at the end of the day all you can really say, we haven't really got any powers to stop this happening, all we can really say is look I think you should go to the police and get an injunction taken out for your own safety and for the safety of your kids. I think they just want to come and open up and tell somebody, just to get it off their chests." (Dr Padden)

This extract demonstrates how healthcare professionals are often frustrated by the interventions which occur with women experiencing domestic violence. Dr Padden does not view the medical encounter, outside of physical injuries, as the appropriate place within which to deal with domestic violence as a social and legal problem. Considering this perception, it is not surprising that Dr Padden finds such interactions frustrating and time-consuming. Doctors can only act on what the patient tells them, or allows them to act on. It is this acknowledgement which has facilitated a shift in the role of healthcare professionals (and doctors in particular) towards a more holistic conception of health which incorporates wider non-medical complaints within medical discourse. As the number of non-medical complaints presented to healthcare professionals increases, doctors are more reliant on the subjective social experience of their patients in order to diagnose and treat specific health-related problems. Research (Peters et al, 1998) has demonstrated that patients themselves are aware of this powerful position, and will use their own knowledge of their health complaint or experience to accept or reject the diagnosis and treatment advocated by healthcare professionals. It could be argued that much of the frustration which healthcare professionals experience in relation to medicalised social problems emanates from the assertion of this power by patients within the medical encounter. It is important, therefore, that the medical model adopted by healthcare professionals continues to alter in relation to shifting organisational structures which emphasise patient power and responsibility over health issues.

Healthcare professionals' perceptions of medical interventions with women presenting with domestic violence-related injuries were often dependent on how the professional perceived their professional role more generally. Those professionals who considered their professional responsibility to be in a constant state of flux which undermined their professionalism were more likely to offer patient-based treatment options of both a medical and non-medical nature. Those healthcare professionals who resisted medicalisation often found medicalised health problems frustrating due to a general disdain about the changing role of the health practitioner. Those healthcare professionals who, while acknowledging the frustrations of medicalisation, accepted this as an historically and culturally specific change in the professionals' role, were more likely to challenge their own preconceived ideas about domestic violence. It is important to note that this type of definition of role was only offered by a minority (four) of the participating healthcare professionals. The personal ideologies which individual health professionals have in relation to specific roles are considered as relevant, not only by contemporary professional bodies (GMC, 1993), in their advocacy of specific types of training models intended to produce more reflexive medics, but also as it forms the basis of medicine within an historical context (Tuckett et al, 1985). These issues will be developed further in Chapter Thirteen, in relation to both community-based health training and inter-agency collaboration.

Counsellors

It became clear through interviews with healthcare professionals and the participating women from stage one that counselling was an important resource utilised in 'domestic violence cases'. The second stage participants included two counsellors located in general practice, and questions were asked of all the healthcare professionals relating to their use of such services. Many of the general practice surgeries where I conducted second stage interviews either had counsellors attached to the surgery or were in the process of implementing such services. These counsellors were perceived as enabling the surgery to deal with low grade mental health problems such as anxiety and depression, which would otherwise take up much of the time of general practitioners who did not feel they had the appropriate skills to deal with such problems effectively, despite having done so for considerable time.

> "We have a counsellor in the practice and we refer a lot of people to her, and I would send to her if I felt there was relationship difficulties or suspected that something was going on and I'm sure that's one area where she would want to treat them as well. We also liaise with the community health team, so sometimes I refer people there if they have a psychiatric need." (Dr Eagland)

> "I think that they [counsellors] might well help these ladies, or men who are victims of domestic violence could be greatly helped by counselling. We are looking with somebody with particular skills in that area." (Dr Fagan)

> "We've got a very high demand for low grade mental health problems, I don't mean things like schizophrenia, pure mental illness which is going to go to the mental heath team anyway, it's the more reactive depressions, marriage problems, not coping, we find that we get absolutely flooded and get miles behind because we're getting endless numbers of tearful women." (Dr Padden)

The importance of counselling has already emerged in many of the extracts from interviews with healthcare professionals, particularly in relation to woman-centred forms of intervention, and issues of disclosure and communication. The extract above from Dr Eagland suggests that it is exactly these types of issues which counsellors want to treat. There is a serious issue about the use of in-house surgery counsellors which will be discussed later in relation to the communication between healthcare professionals more generally; it is relevant, however, that the counsellors who were interviewed in this research were extremely concerned at what they saw as a 'dustbin' syndrome, where they were being used to deal with all the issues that medical personnel felt uncomfortable dealing with. Identifying and utilising counselling as an appropriate treatment option for women experiencing domestic violence is positive, as it represents a move away from the use of antidepressants and tranquillisers to manage psychosomatic injuries. Such alternatives are not, however, unproblematic. As discussed in Chapter Four, there were instances where the participating women felt unable to talk to a counsellor, were unable to afford counselling, or perceived the relatively short duration representative of a lack of concern. It was also suggested earlier that, rather than professional counselling, the presenting women want validation of their experiences.

There is also growing concern (Schornstein, 1997; Gondolf, 1998) about the use of joint counselling in domestic violence cases. This was evident both in this research and in responses to the domestic violence and health questionnaire (Abbott and Williamson, 1999), where 52.3% of respondents believed suggesting both partners receive counselling to be good advice to women experiencing domestic violence. This practice is both dangerous, in relation to the woman being punished for disclosing the occurrence of violence, and counterproductive. Joint counselling can only work as a treatment alternative if both parties are able to communicate their problems with one another. The power dynamics and issues of control so obviously relevant within a domestically violent situation make such a prerequisite impossible. Health practitioners should be aware of the possible dangers associated with advocating joint counselling, and avoid it wherever possible.

Prescribing antidepressants

In relation to suicides and para-suicidal activity, general practitioners do still utilise drugs to control 'low grade' mental health problems, and are often aware of the problems of doing so.

> "Yes, well it's a multi-pronged treatment in that there are multiple treatment options. I use antidepressants and medication a lot for

people having mental health problems related to family problems because I think that if the counselling is gonna help and the drugs are gonna help I don't see why they shouldn't have them both at the same time. I go for the whole lot if it's going to work. I think I probably over-medicalise sometimes but then if they don't want the medication they generally come back and tell me that they don't."
(Dr Eagland)

Dr Eagland is aware of the problems relating to the prescription of antidepressant drugs, as has been documented in existing literature (Stark and Flitcraft, 1982, 1995, 1996; Klingbeil and Boyd, 1984; Easteal and Easteal, 1992). However, while Dr Eagland identifies that many women may return because they do not want to take drugs, she does not acknowledge that there are serious implications in prescribing drugs to a group of women who are statistically more likely to attempt suicide than the general population (Stark and Flitcraft, 1995, 1996). This was evident in the assertions of Debbie and Iris in Chapter Four.

Despite the reluctance of many healthcare professionals to accept that para-suicides are a very real health problem related to the experience of domestic violence, I asked all the healthcare professionals to identify how they would deal with para-suicides when they received notification from a casualty department that a patient had been admitted following a suicide attempt. The following extracts detail the responses of some of the respondents.

[In relation to suicides and reaction of health visitor] "To be honest, who would look after the children. It depends on the age of the child too because it's fairly easy, in inverted commas, if the child is under one and the mum is doing this as we have direct access then to the mother and baby unit at the ... hospital, but I think we would consider that she needed expert help of some kind? I would certainly be referring to the GP in the hope that the mental health team would be involved if they weren't already and then our role in that would be to keep visiting and keep supporting but we would want more expert help than ourselves. Work together hopefully." (Ms Lacey)

As with earlier extracts from the interview with Ms Lacey, she is reluctant to acknowledge her own power as a healthcare professional, and undermines her knowledge and impact within the health interaction in relation to a medical hierarchy where others have more power than herself. Also, we can observe the differentiation which occurs between different types of familial abuse where Ms Lacey perceives her role to be concerned with the welfare and provision of services related to children. She does, however, advocate an inter-agency health response, which is positive, and which will be considered in more detail in Chapter Twelve.

"Well this is the 64 million dollar question, para-suicide, because of course you've got to know about it first of all before you can do anything and you don't always know about it. If it comes to your attention then the big worry is that people who persistently self-harm, whether or not their intention is to kill themselves, eventually sometimes do. So whether your intention is to call attention to yourself, or kill yourself if you keep doing it long enough you will eventually die at your own hands so it is a worry, but you asked me how I deal with it, I deal with it by asking them to confront what they're doing and is it the best way of dealing with their situation and asking them whether self-mutilation is actually going to achieve anything. But for a lot of people, inarticulate people, who feel trapped, they don't see any other way of dealing with it, so what you don't want to do is remove their prop and not replace it with something else, or remove their coping mechanism and not replace it with something else. So if somebody walked in right now and said 'I took an overdose last week and the week before', ok, what would I do? I suppose I would try and use a cognitive approach to find out exactly what they think they're achieving, why they're doing what they're doing, there's a better way. Try and exchange what I perceive as their inappropriate response to something more productive, if that was possible, that would be my approach." (Dr Gabb)

Dr Gabb's response to my question about para-suicide demonstrates a thorough understanding of the problems and frustrations inherent in dealing with women who consistently self-harm, including para-suicidal activity. Dr Gabb's suggestion that it is necessary to challenge an inappropriate response by suggesting more productive behaviour is progressive, and would assist a woman who engages in such behaviour as a result of domestic violence. The only cause for concern in the above extract is the suggestion that it is inarticulate patients who indulge in self-harming behaviour. This identifies types of patients who articulate themselves in this manner, rather than demonstrating an understanding that experiencing domestic violence results in the silencing of the majority of its 'victims'. Dr Gabb's response, however, came closest to acknowledging the psychological findings of this research, which has examined how women who experience domestic violence negotiate their psychological injuries.

> "It always means you have got to wonder whether the next time they will be successful, because you see I am not there, you are not there as a guardian angel, you are only there as a support, you would like to be a guardian angel, but you can't take all these women home. You can't take them all home and be the guardian angel and watch over them, you have to make a decision, is this woman really suicidal?, or is she para-suicidal? If she is only para-suicidal is it reasonable to see her today and see her again in a week's time? Is it reasonable to give her supportive medication for those so many days, so many days could be expensive if you are only giving her seven days medication, can you really afford to give her twenty eight days, and if she is suicidal is it appropriate to get a psychiatrist involved today, or let it wait until next time, because you think that it is the first time that it has been discussed?" (Dr Habberley)

Dr Habberley's response is particularly interesting, as he introduces the concept of cost. He also clearly distinguishes between suicidal and para-suicidal behaviour. While such a distinction is valid, considering the motivations behind the para-suicidal activity of women experiencing domestic violence, to distinguish between the seriousness of each is not useful, as it creates a hierarchy of motivation. As both Dr Habberley and Dr Gabb have acknowledged, there is a very real possibility that para-suicidal behaviour will ultimately result in suicide. Considering these assertions in the context of comments made by stage one participants in Chapter Three, it is pertinent to ask a number of questions. First, why are women's requests for help not heeded earlier, before psychological injuries manifest themselves in para-suicidal activity? The participating women discussed seeking validation of their experiences and the non-physical injuries they sustained in health interactions which took place prior to their para-suicidal activities. Second, it is pertinent to ask why women's para-suicidal activity is not taken seriously, when subsequent attempts could be successful.

Dr Habberley also acknowledges the frustrations which dealing with para-suicidal patients elicit, in that an individual healthcare professional cannot act as a patient's guardian angel. While this is true of all professionals dealing with domestic violence, it would be pertinent, in the hypothetical situation Dr Habberley describes, to refer such a patient to specialised service providers with extensive experience of dealing with women recovering from the soul-destroying effects of domestic violence. The reasons why healthcare professionals are reluctant to refer patients directly to voluntary services will be addressed in Chapter Twelve, in relation to general referrals to other health and statutory service providers. Despite the reluctance of healthcare professionals to make the connection between para-suicide and domestic violence, it is clear from the above extracts that para-suicide is a problem, particularly among the female patient population. This contradiction is worrying, as it suggests that healthcare professionals are not taking seriously research statistics which identify a connection between domestic violence and suicide, particularly in relation to their prescription of antidepressant drugs.

This chapter has identified how healthcare professionals are competent at identifying physical injuries, and in some cases psychosomatic ones. The reluctance of practitioners to acknowledge the domestic violence origins of para-suicide is worrying but consistent with international research which has examined domestic violence and health. The responses discussed above concern individual practitioners. As demonstrated in Chapter Five, women who experience domestic violence engage in a diverse range of help-seeking activities. This implies that communication between practitioners is important, beyond individual interactions. The following chapter addresses this problem by examining documentation and the naming of domestic violence.

Notes

[1] These categories are not exclusive.

[2] These categories are not exclusive.

TEN

Documentation and naming

This chapter is concerned with the issue of documentation, which was an area of concern in the stage one interviews, as discussed in Chapter Four. Examining the issues of culpability, documentation, confidentiality, and the medical record is important, as it is through the written patient record that medical complaints become integrated in medical discourse, through research and the acknowledgement of clinical practice. There are a number of issues which relate both directly and indirectly to the use of medical records, including the use of medical records in training; legal discourses; as an 'event' itself within the medical encounter; as representative of the hierarchy which exists between different healthcare professionals; naming; recording; and the appropriation of the sick role. Examining the medical record is important, as it has been suggested (Berg, 1996) that the medical record, rather than merely representing the medical encounter, is an event in itself. This implies that the medical record, like the appropriation of the sick role, exerts a social control function, situated between the medical encounter and medical discourse. Considering that medical records document the medical encounter and the processes, diagnosis, and treatments utilised within it, it is frequently used in research to ascertain the health needs and provision of local communities and society more generally. The medical record functions, therefore, to legitimise the entrance of knowledge into medical discourse, and as a result is important in the evaluation of the health interaction which occurs between women who experience domestic violence and healthcare professionals.

The medical record as a legal document

The most formidable function of the medical record is in legal discourse. Due to the position of medical discourse in society, such records are considered valuable as accurate representations of individuals' experiences of health and well-being, particularly in relation to crimes against the person. First, considering the assertion that the medical record is an event in itself rather than a representation of the medical encounter (Berg, 1996), this could be questioned. Second, problems exist in identifying specific aspects of medicalised problems such as domestic violence, as documented throughout this book. When discussing the use of the medical record, particularly in relation to domestic violence-related injuries, the assertions by the stage two participants demonstrated how they considered the legal implications of their 'aid memoir' to be of central importance. In North America, healthcare professionals (and psychiatrists in particular) have, in some US states, been required by law to advise other professionals when so-called 'vulnerable adults' who are at risk from domestic violence present with domestic violence-related injuries. The problematic nature of such laws and protocols are well documented (Sanders and Sheva, 1995; Sonkin, 1986) and it is unlikely that we will see the emergence of similar laws in Britain. However, such a law does highlight the responsibility of professionals generally to address issues of violence where the life or health of a patient may be at risk. The medical record is particularly important for professionals to document their own behaviour and interaction so as to protect their own reputation and professionalism:

> "I think there is a general rule of thumb – as accurately as possible really. Certainly making sure that things like dates, times are clearly documented. Write down what the patient actually said was the cause and particularly with physical violence, write down what the patient said as far as mental or physical violence was concerned, who by, in the situation. I'd certainly cover myself I'm afraid to say by writing down that I've suggested or recommended that they see the police or to protect themselves because at the end of the day if this happens again and someone goes home and is killed by their partner ... obviously if there are physical signs that's got to be documented graphically ... I think the more detail the better generally."
> (Dr Padden)

While the term of reference Dr Padden utilises (rule of thumb) is extremely unfortunate (due to the historical significance of this legislation[1] in relation to the legal advocacy of domestic violence), his assertion that "the more detail the better generally" is something which many of the healthcare professionals I interviewed advocated in theory, but in practice were unable to deliver. This was due to a number of reasons, the most frequently mentioned being time restraints within the consultation period. Second, problems with documentation existed due to healthcare professionals' own unease in dealing with domestic violence generally, and third, due to the reluctance of healthcare professions to name domestic violence for fear of legitimising it as a valid health complaint. While it is unlikely that healthcare professionals would be prosecuted for failing to document the existence of domestic violence, since women who experience domestic violence are adults, the example of the Vulnerable Adults Act cited above does question the legal culpability of healthcare professionals in relation to their use of the medical record. A number of women who participated in this research were extremely disappointed that their medical records did not contain information about their previous abuse. While the legal position of these omissions would be fragile, it is feasible that failing to document suspicions of domestic violence contravenes medical ethics codes (Amnesty International, 1994) as well as professional guidelines (GMC, 1993), if not legal ones. On a more practical note, such omissions also make it difficult to evaluate the prevalence and specific health needs of women experiencing domestic violence[2].

The response of healthcare professionals to concerns raised about documentation by the participating women was again contradictory. Some would always record domestic violence injuries so that the information would be available for criminal proceedings, whereas others made a distinction between general patient notes and forensic notes which were requested specifically for legal purposes.

"There are three sorts of recording: there is mental recording, which is truly what the patient tells you, it is probably not appropriate to write on paper. We use the written word, mark one pencil is wonderful, it doesn't go off-line, it doesn't get itself wrong and it tends to work. Computers tend to go off-line, and get hung and they are very temperamental. You may in a situation in here you would probably put an entry, you could probably put something like assault. It says no more, on the menu, and on the written word we are going to have to put the incident with a list of the injuries, those seen and those, pain can be described, told where it is but you may not have seen the injury, but you have to record it. So a good record of the statement of what a patient says, the facts, and your own observations. Because some day I may have to stand up in a court of law and say it says, or the patient says." (Dr Habberley)

This extract from Dr Habberley questions the usefulness and scope of technologies used to record patient consultations. He clearly suggests that categories exist within the computer software which alter the definitions available to explain the cause of an injury. In this case he suggests that he would probably utilise 'assault', as domestic violence is not an option within such software. While new technologies may assist healthcare professionals, their limitations should also be considered. Dr Habberley also raises questions about the validity of the experiences women who present with domestic violence-related injuries disclose. While he does not personally doubt such experiences – Dr Habberley had a particularly flexible view of the medical encounter and his social and professional responsibility on a number of issues including domestic violence – he is clearly wary of recording information without question, due to his own culpability should that information be required for legal reasons.

> "In common I would have to say our notes are not always detailed enough but again it would depend on how it came up. If they walked in and explicitly say 'The police have told me to come', then you're very careful, you write 'a three by two centimetre yellowish bruise on the right hand forehead consistent with the story of whatever, bruised ribs...' and you detail in great depth exactly what's what and how long the cuts are and some opinion as well as to whether it's possible that this injury could have been sustained from the story that was given. But if you're in a position where this is a depressed patient who keeps coming to you because they're depressed and during counselling it comes out that she's subject to this it would be very unlikely I'd start describing lesions, but I'd still make a definite record that this is what the story was." (Dr Gabb)

Dr Aaron made a distinction between medical and forensic notes. He stated that he wouldn't record forensic notes unless specifically asked to do so. This was due to too much pressure; instead he would make a quick reference. This differentiation in medical recording was dependent on distinguishing between medical reasons to make the record and medical-legal reasons to make records. Used example of road traffic accidents where would ask if patient intended to take further action which would then alter types of notes taken. (Dr Aaron)

Both Dr Gabb and Dr Aaron distinguish between types of documentation in the medical record, which relates to the likelihood of such information being required for legal purposes. The differentiation which Dr Gabb makes in reference to physical and non-physical injuries is particularly disconcerting, as it is frequently non-physical abuses which are difficult to prove and prosecute, whether supported by medical documentation or not. Patients experiencing domestic violence may be reluctant to request that forensic notes be made relating to their domestic violence-related injuries when they are already reluctant to admit that domestic violence is the cause of an injury. Healthcare professionals must ensure, therefore, that if they are making a distinction between medical and forensic notes that this decision is not always based on the request of the patient, particularly where domestic violence is the cause of injury and where the patient is likely to be still living in a domestically violent situation with the abuser.

Confidentiality

One issue frequently cited in relation to medical records is confidentiality. In the interviews with the participating women from stage one, the issue of confidentiality arose only in terms of the need to ensure that the perpetrator of the violence was not aware they had disclosed the occurrence of violence to a third party. In many cases they had disclosed to a healthcare professional because of the confidentiality of the medical consultation. This in itself can cause problems, particularly if a healthcare professional feels they cannot discuss the case with other members of their primary healthcare team because their colleagues have contact with the family as a whole, or if the surgery is large and a diverse range of healthcare professionals have access to medical records and/or patient notes. The issue of confidentiality exists, therefore, not in isolation, but in conjunction with the issue of communication with other colleagues and the medical record itself.

> "The way we do things I'd put headings on the computer and I'd probably not actually put that on the computer, probably just put it in the notes ... the computer is to easy to get to, people prescribing, letters for this that and the other ... also it's quite a small community, a lot of members of staff are involved with the patients, friends and you've just got to add that little extra caution really." (Dr Padden)

> "I think that it is very important that you alert your colleagues to tactful issues. If the patient objects to what is in their medical record they can object at anytime that it is given to another third party. For instance, insurance companies write for reports on patients' entitlement to reform, if I suspected that their lifestyle would put them at risk of HIV I would probably suggest that the patient saw

the report beforehand, if they did not wish that to be known then they could say so, but then you have to mark the report has been altered because the patient asked them to. A very difficult situation."
(Dr Fagan)

The comments made in the above extracts demonstrate the contradictions of confidentiality in the medical record. Comparing the assertions made by Dr Padden and Dr Fagan, who work in the same general practice surgery, demonstrates that while Dr Padden is reluctant to use the medical record because of the number of people who have access to it within the surgery, that is exactly the same reason why Dr Fagan would utilise the medical record. Also an issue in the extract from Dr Fagan is the way in which the medical record can be utilised to document the life-styles of patients. This is important, as the example Dr Fagan gives relates to the functioning of capitalism, where the medical practitioner is making health and life-style judgments on behalf of financial institutions, who can marginalise and/or exclude specific individuals and groups of individuals. The perceptions of the participating women in relation to the control function of the medical record will be examined shortly. The issue of confidentiality is, however, very serious, particularly in relation to the use of information technologies which are intended to make the medical intervention more productive. Such technologies, while they may enable other health professionals to access information about other services (for example, for repeat prescriptions, referrals, or laboratory test results), and thus give general practitioners more time for other consultations, become unproductive if they result in the medical record not being used to record sensitive issues which may be central to a patient's medical history. The importance of bibliographic material in the diagnosis of a patient's injuries has been documented generally (Grant et al, 1994) and in relation to domestic violence (Klingbeil and Boyd, 1984). If such material is being omitted due to fears about confidentiality, then there are serious doubts about the adequacy of such technological aids (Kinkhorst et al, 1996). The issue of confidentiality within medical discourse has itself resulted in delays in the implementation of technological aids intended to improve communication between healthcare professionals (Wyatt, 1998), particularly between primary and secondary service providers.

The medical record and the medical hierarchy

The following extract from Ms Lacey illustrates some of the issues concerning different types of medical records and patient notes as utilised by different healthcare professionals.

"Other health visitors and perhaps the management, the only other people who do have access to them eventually will be the school health people, school health doctors, paediatricians, the clinical medical officers they used to call them, the child health doctors would if you referred the child for some reason, or some assessment or weren't happy about with the development or something, they would see those other records that say this is what the home situation is like. Technically speaking the GP could and social services have sometimes but I have made the clients aware, the occasion I'm thinking of was something that the client had disclosed anyway and was perfectly well aware that I was going to take that to social services, but very rarely and other than that no." (Ms Lacey)

An important revelation in the above extract is that while general practitioners may be sensitive about the medical records they keep, it is common practice for the family histories and patient/family notes of health visitors to be available for the inspection of other health professionals, and in some cases social workers, teachers and so on. These discrepancies between the status of patient notes in the various health professions, while representative of the hierarchised nature of the medical profession as a whole, highlight issues around professional ideologies, professional status and autonomy. The professional respect of those located within the medical hierarchy as superior to others is translated in practice as enabling them to expect autonomy within their work, while not in the work of others. The issue of confidentiality highlights the contradictions between requiring supportive and collaborative relationships with one's colleagues, and other healthcare professionals, while also attempting to maintain a degree of autonomy with which to strengthen the boundaries of one's professionalism. The positions taken on this issue by the participating healthcare professionals depended on whether they saw their role within the strictly defined boundaries of the medical profession in isolation or in conjunction with other medical and non-medical social services. Those who adopted a purely medical definition of their roles were more likely to see the issue of confidentiality as a significant part of their professionalism, whereas those whose definition was more socially, culturally or philosophically based were more likely to perceive their professional role in relation to, and therefore dependent on, the professional roles and experiences of others.

> "The way I look at it. The medical record is a confidential document. So if I accept that then I have to accept that it's safe to write anything in it, insurance reports, access to information for future adoption or fostering medicals, they all can see that information, the decision will be whether to disclose at that point what's in the notes, whether it's relevant to a situation. I don't think there's anything to be gained from hiding information that someone is suffering." (Dr Gabb)

The extract above from Dr Gabb is included as an example of good practice. While it acknowledges the role healthcare professionals have in the selective dissemination of confidential notes, it also acknowledges that the role of the healthcare professional functions in conjunction with the roles of other professionals within society. Acknowledging the location of medical discourse within wider society may not appear particularly progressive, but it was not a perspective evident in the majority of the second stage interviews.

The medical record, as an integral part of the medical encounter, clearly perpetuates the professional boundaries of different health professionals within the medical hierarchy. This is evident in the different ways in which nurses and doctors, for example, use the medical record to document their work and patient care. In secondary service provision in particular, nurses' documentation is frequently restricted to routine measurements and the implementation of doctors' treatments (Berg, 1996). This is in comparison to the use of the medical record by doctors, who are able to extend their medical gaze beyond their specific interactions with patients. As such, it has been suggested that "the record enters into the (re)production of hierarchical relations at the same time as it affords the creation of a manageable patient's body" (Berg, 1996, p 513).

Just as general practitioners considered the categorisations of injuries in hospital 'flimsies' to be inadequate and vague (this will be discussed in more detail in relation to inter-agency collaboration in Chapter Twelve), so too are the references to domestic violence in the general practitioners' own medical records. The historic relationship between secondary service providers and primary healthcare teams often makes communication and collaboration difficult (Walker, 1988). This problem, it has been suggested (Marshall, 1998), is exacerbated by the move by general practitioners in particular to assert their own "unique identity" in opposition to traditionally hospital specialist-based secondary provision. The medical record has been investigated (Marshall, 1998) as a possible training tool with which to facilitate further collaborations between general practitioners and specialists. While general practitioners thought that such clinically-based training might be useful, researchers found that specialists were uncomfortable using individual patient cases to facilitate training. This is partly exacerbated by the role of general practitioners as consumers of specialist secondary service provision. As this example demonstrates, communication between different healthcare professionals through medical documentation is problematised by both the historic and the market-driven relationship which currently exists between such professionals. This example highlights once again the position of domestic violence in a range of medical debates.

Patients' access to medical records

The issue of patients having access to their medical records was introduced earlier in relation to the experiences of Carol, one of the stage one participants. She was concerned that her medical record did not include references to a number of years of violence and abuse which had resulted in physical and non-physical injuries. It was interesting, therefore, that the access which patients have to medical records was one of the reasons given by healthcare professionals for their reluctance to explicitly record domestic violence.

> "Well I think I would write down that I suspect that she must be a victim of violence. I would do that because I consider the medical record to be not only my aid memoir but it is important what my partners know what I am thinking in case they see it, so that if I am on holiday and a crisis occurs. It is not derogatory to the woman, it is relevant to her condition and it is important that suspicions are known and put it down clearly in the record what you think has gone on. Records are confidential and people do have access to them since 1991 so I am going to write in the record the facts, not my opinion which might be 'I think the silly tart has asked for it'." (Dr Fagan)

Dr Fagan, while aware of the stigma which women who experience domestic violence suffer, suggests that recording information is vital, both in terms of the work of his colleagues and in the treatment of the patients' 'condition'. He also refers to the issue of patient access to medical records, and suggests that patient access influences the way in which he documents a patient's injuries. Having access to medical records is important, therefore, in relation to issues of control. If a patient is denied access, or does not even know she is entitled to such information, she cannot fully participate in the medical interaction, either on a first or subsequent consultation. This has important ramifications for the differentiation of responsibility between the patient and healthcare professional within the medical interaction. While health practitioners may advocate patient responsibility for health, such a position is contradictory unless they are willing to negotiate power and control within the medical discourse. This is a particularly pertinent point in relation to domestic violence.

> "No, I don't record on written at all actually. When they're sitting here, they either sit there or there and they can see the screen and they can see what I write, and if they object they object. But they see what's written so ... nobody has said 'no sorry I don't want that on', it's just gone on either as marital disharmony, or domestic whatever ... and the facts, because I think the point where people do come, I'd like to think they come for support and all the other things but there's also an advantage of them coming to the doctor because there's this sort of status that we have in society that if it went to court, if there were things then it would, it could, the doctor may be expected to report, or they'd want the doctor as an ally on their side, so it makes it sometimes difficult if you're dealing with both halves." (Dr Jabber)

Dr Jabber's comments are relevant to this discussion, as not only does he acknowledge the social position and professional status of healthcare professionals, but he demonstrates a problem which was inherent in a number of second stage interviews relating to naming.

Naming

Healthcare professionals seemed reluctant to use the term domestic violence when discussing documentation, despite using it throughout the interview process, and despite the majority being able to clearly define the term. When discussing a permanent record of the medical interaction, healthcare professionals referred to 'family problems', 'problems at home', 'marital disharmony' or 'domestic whatever...' as in the above extract. The importance of naming has already been acknowledged in this book, as have the connotations of a variety of terms used to describe the experience of domestic violence (see Chapter One). Naming through diagnosis also relates specifically to the appropriation of the sick role. Research (Peters et al, 1998) has identified that the fears and anxieties patients often have in relation to their health complaint and/or the medical encounter itself are often removed when their ill health is named through diagnosis. Naming the experience of domestic violence serves to validate the subjective experience of domestic violence while simultaneously legitimating the sick role appropriation of individual patients. The reluctance of healthcare professionals to name domestic violence is not surprising considering the wider difficulties they have in dealing with domestic violence. While healthcare professionals interact with women experiencing domestic violence in their clinical practice, they are reluctant to document a problem which they find frustrating and which would be legitimated through the documentation process. The contradictions inherent in the medicalisation debate are particularly relevant to domestic violence. It is not accidental that, despite treating women who experience domestic violence, healthcare professionals are reluctant to name that experience in medical diagnoses and documentation. This is a process which, while it has been suggested it would depoliticise women's anger and experience (Illich, 1976; Riessman, 1983), would also legitimise women's experiences as valid within a discourse which has a great deal of social power. It is important to acknowledge, particularly in relation to the medical record, that while healthcare professionals may deny the subjective experience of patients through the diagnosis and naming of specific complaints according to a biomedical model of healthcare, healthcare professionals also deny their own subjective experiences in such a process. This was most evident within this research in terms of the different boundaries set by both research participant groups (Williamson, 1999, 2000). It could also be suggested that the shift from a biomedical to an holistic model of healthcare emanates partly from healthcare professionals' unease at denying their own subjectivity in relation to an increasing number of medicalised health problems.

> "We all work differently, I always make it quite plain that there are two sets of records kept about the family, one is the child's record, the red book, and I'd be very careful and I do point out that I will be very careful what I put in that because although domestic violence and what is going on in the home, the situation is important to the

child, this is the sort of book that the doctor, the dentist, granny and all sorts of people can be reading and I think the effects for the child of what you're recording there, I mean advice you've given for the child. And I always make it quite plain on the first visit that I will keep a separate family care record because I want to know about mum's health and the family situation and the kind of support network she's got. So I suppose I take it for granted then that they know that I am going to record something about them or their situation. If I suspected some kind of abuse was going on but didn't actually have her saying there was then I think I would be recording the symptoms, if you know what I mean, I would be very careful to say in terms 'I am not happy because', not in so many words but the recording of the visit wouldn't say 'mother well', just because mum said she was, I would be very specific about 'Mum reported that she was fine, but she looked tired, or drawn or tense or did this or said that', so I wouldn't actually put my opinion in there, I wouldn't actually say 'I think this is going on', but I would put 'This is what I've seen and this is what I've heard and I'm not happy in some way', and then hopefully, because I think that you need a reminder when you go back again next time you need to say no, no three, four, five weeks on the run now this woman's looked like this and said it's just a cold." (Ms Lacey)

As a health visitor Ms Lacey is required to keep detailed case notes and family histories which can be accessed by those healthcare professionals placed higher in the medical hierarchy. As such, it is not surprising that Ms Lacey, like the general practitioners quoted above, is reluctant to document domestic violence and therefore acknowledge the experiences of women who suffer from it. While recording domestic violence in vague terms is an improvement from those who are reluctant to record domestic violence at all, it is still extremely confusing, particularly if we are to rely on medical records to identify the occurrence of domestic violence on a wider scale (Grant et al, 1994).

Documenting non-physical injuries

The results of misreporting and misdiagnosis in relation to domestic violence generally have been well documented in literature from North America (Goldberg and Tomlanovich, 1984; Klingbeil and Boyd, 1984); if we are to avoid the same problems within Britain then we must begin to acknowledge the occurrence of domestic violence and record our suspicions as such. Some of the problems seem to arise when making notes about non-physical injuries, the cause of which cannot be so easily verified. Again this is problematic, particularly if healthcare professionals are prepared to acknowledge that psychosomatic non-physical injuries are, in some cases, caused by domestic violence but are not recorded as such.

> "In non-physical injuries you are actually saying what the patient tells you. He ignores me, or he goes to the pub every night and comes home, or as a patient said to me this morning she didn't come back last night and I sat up in a chair all night and she didn't come home this morning before I came to see you in surgery. This particular woman knows that she is causing her husband worry, a form of abuse, call it what you will, but it was written because I need to keep an eye on the chap, to remind myself what is going on." (Dr Habberley)

> "Well, I mean if a woman comes in and makes a statement then you have got a disclosure and you have to document it. If you feel that they are making something up you can put a query violence, it means that your main observation may not be confirmed." (Dr Habberley)

There are many problems which exist at present between the expectations of women presenting with domestic violence-related injuries and the practice of healthcare professionals, particularly concerning the medical record, which may be the only official record that domestic violence is present and that a crime has or is being committed. While recording domestic violence adequately may require the more widespread use of time-consuming forensic notes, tools do exist with which to reduce the administrative workloads involved. These are addressed in Part Three, alongside other practical ways in which to improve the health interaction between healthcare professionals and women who experience domestic violence. No amount of assessment tools, however, will improve the underlying problem of practitioners who are reluctant to name domestic violence as a result of their own unease with the issue generally. This requires more training in dealing with domestic violence, which addresses not only clinical concerns but the wider social and political dynamics of abuse. As a result, Part Three also addresses the issue of training.

Notes

[1] In England, once a woman became a wife, she abdicated any independent claim to be whatever property she had, right up until the Married Women's Property Act of 1895. She also gave up a number of other rights she had as a single woman, and gave her husband the right to inflict corporal punishment upon her (Manoa, 1986, p 148).

[2] Research which has examined medical records in relation to domestic violence includes Stanko et al (1998) and Stark and Flitcraft (1982, 1995, 1996). Such research has had to take into account the reluctance of healthcare professionals to address issues of domestic violence explicitly in the medical record.

Summary to Part Two

This section has highlighted the responses of healthcare professionals to domestic violence. By examining both knowledge and clinical experience of domestic violence it has identified several key points which relate to both bad and good practice. This summary is therefore represented as a list of points which healthcare professionals need to address.

Box 9: Key recommendations and examples of good practice

Healthcare professionals should:

- Be able to define domestic violence.

- Work to policies and guidelines which would assist practitioners in offering a more consistent service to those experiencing domestic violence (see Chapter One for references).

- Have an understanding of their own professional roles and responsibilities and how issues such as domestic violence impact on them.

- Be aware of the constraints and potential within the roles and responsibilities of 'other' medical and non-medical health staff.

- Avoid differentiating between those who experience violence and themselves.

- Be aware that 'blaming victims for staying' is a common but unhelpful reaction.

- Avoid assuming that 'cycle of abuse' and 'dysfunctional family' theories are adequate explanations for violence.

- Locate their practice within a domestic violence discourse. Healthcare professionals' interactions are perceived in relation to wider experiences of abuse, which they cannot control. Ensure their practice does not perpetuate abusive power dynamics.

- Consider the impact of psychosomatic and non-physical injuries in all encounters with women experiencing domestic violence.

- Recognise the existence of the complex post-traumatic stress disorder (PTSD).

- Be aware that some psychological complaints can be confused with complex PTSD.

- Have an understanding of how medical discourse locates women who consistently engage with para-suicidal activity. Be aware of the reasons why domestic violence may impact on this behaviour.

- Consider para-suicidal activity in relation to the biomedical/holistic dichotomy within health interactions. Women may engage in this behaviour because they feel their experiences are not validated within an holistic framework.

- Examine their previous practice to identify the types of treatments they use routinely with possible domestic violence cases.

- Have adequate knowledge to effectively provide such treatments. This is particularly relevant in relation to giving information, advice, and offering broad-based counselling or a 'sympathetic ear'.

- Ensure that women remain in control of treatments and do not feel further disempowered or isolated.

- Offer a range of treatments, which may include doing nothing but leaving a patient's options to return open.

- Name domestic violence.

- Record domestic violence. Particularly non-physical injuries.

- Tell patients that they are recording domestic violence for future reference, or that the patient can have access to records privately.

- Ensure that communication between health professionals is followed up.

- Check that computer packages enable them to record domestic violence.

- Ensure that health teams are using records in a consistent manner.

- Communicate with their colleagues. This gives them support which reduces frustration and ensures that the potential for others to intervene is achieved.

- NEVER blame women for the violence they experience. Such views will further isolate patients from help, by undermining their self-esteem and reinforcing the assertions of the perpetrator.

- Consider their social responsibilities to address this issue. This is not merely a health issue but has wider ramifications for society as a whole. Healthcare professionals have a part to play in the dissemination of ideologies that reinforce the argument that the actions of domestic violence perpetrators are criminal and unacceptable.

Part Three:
Clinicians' training and inter-agency collaboration

The issue of collaboration both within and beyond the health professions has arisen throughout this book, in relation to specific interactions, as well as to wider inter-agency collaborations between groups with different professional statuses. The following chapters address these issues, as it is imperative that any approach to tackling domestic violence in relation to health occurs in a context where a range of professions are involved. For example, the discrepancy between the relative power of general practitioners and health visitors has already arisen, and is, it could be suggested, a barrier to more effective interventions with women who present with domestic violence-related injuries. The concept of inter-agency work and the impact it has on the professional identities, and clinical practice, of a range of professional groups also has massive implications for training. The concept of training has therefore been included in this section, as it represents where professional identities are learned, as well as an area where examples of good practice and information can be disseminated.

Part Three will begin by examining the collaboration and communication which exists between healthcare professionals. Second, it will look at inter-agency work beyond the medical professions, and finally, it will examine training in relation to community training models, which represent a shift away from biomedical/wound-led models of health and embody changing concepts of learning and of interventions in domestic violence. This final section will also introduce a number of training tools which would be useful for training healthcare professionals about domestic violence. An inter-agency focus is assumed, as the extracts included in Part One illustrated how the participating women from stage one considered their interactions with health professionals in the context of their wider help-seeking activities. Any training tools adopted for health professionals must ensure, therefore, that they do not perpetuate concepts of professionalism which preclude inter-agency collaboration.

ELEVEN

Intra-professional collaboration and communication

A number of issues have already been raised by both participant groups about the communication which occurs between health professionals. These include: communication between primary and secondary services; different members of the individual primary practice surgeries; and issues related to the professional roles of different health practitioners. This chapter addresses these issues, as it is important to contextualise and understand the complexity of the medical professions before looking at collaboration beyond these professional groups in light of multi-agency initiatives. This chapter will address the relative positions of health visitors, nurses and female general practitioners, and the communication across primary and secondary service providers, in order to identify issues which arise as a result of the differentiation of professional responsibilities. The historical emergence of different health professionals has defined many of the boundaries which currently exist between specific practitioners. It should also be acknowledged that, due to the impact of socially caused ill health, many of these boundaries are shifting as a result of the so-called 'health crisis'. The following discussions should be considered, therefore, as grounded in these contemporary changes.

Health visitors and practice nurses

The following extracts come from one of the interviewed health visitors, and relate to her experiences of working with practice nurses, other health visitors and general practitioners.

> "I think it helps if you've got a peer group support as well, if you can go back to the office and say 'I really mishandled that, what do you reckon I could do to make amends', and then you can go back with confidence and say 'I think the last time we met you were trying to tell me something about … and I'm sorry I wasn't receptive but …' or, 'Would you like to tell me more about such and such?', I think that's something I find very difficult with health visiting at the

moment. We used to have a lovely support group together, based here, there were always five of us likely to be around when you came back to the office and you can say 'Oh I don't know' and you can bounce ideas off people and you come back with 'Well maybe it's not that disastrous after all, don't do yourself down, you can go back and do, and pick it up', because you always can can't you? And it's never that, not really ever that emergency, not in health visiting usually anyway that you couldn't go back next week or whatever and the situation's pretty much the same. I think we've now got fragmented: there are people who are just one or two or maybe three in a surgery now." (Ms Lacey)

"You could get support from the practice nurses in that you could discuss the family with them and they will probably know that family because they will have been doing the baby's injections or whatever." (Ms Lacey)

Considering the frustrations and difficulties faced when dealing with patients presenting with domestic violence-related injuries, the ability of healthcare professionals to support and assist one another is particularly important, as is being able to communicate and develop supportive relationships with non-medical professionals such as social workers, the police, teachers and so on. The environment which Ms Lacey identifies, where she was surrounded in the office by other health visitors, has disappeared due to funding restrictions and the restructuring of healthcare provision. This restructuring process, while it may have been necessary due to funding restrictions, does not acknowledge the importance of support networks and inter-professional communications, and does not offer alternative support networks with which to replace those that have been lost. This lack of control over one's work environment can be attributed to the power which a professional group holds, and non-medical personnel appear to have very little power in this respect. It is also interesting that Ms Lacey identifies practice nurses and other health visitors as supportive, considering the hierarchical nature of healthcare as a whole. This is evident in the assertions Ms Lacey made earlier, in relation to her perceived lack of knowledge and influence in the medical interaction as a whole. The extracts above also imply that, while other health visitors and practice nurses may be available sources of support and advice due to their comparative position on the medical hierarchy, other more powerful health practitioners are not considered as an adequate professional resource.

"GPs, bless them, it depends on the nature of the beast I'm afraid because there's certainly one where I've tried to say, the lady with the broken ribs did actually try to talk to the GP about her mental state and the fact that she was actually disclosing feelings of suicidal feelings, self-harm, those sorts of feelings and was very very depressed and in this situation which I was not happy about at all, not for her sake, or for the children's sake and I tried to talk over with him the difficulties and he put his coat on and was walking through the door 'Yes, yes, yes I'll go and see her', so that isn't very supportive. But then there are other GPs that I feel caught at the right moment, you could discuss them and you could, but I feel now it's very new being in the surgery and it's fairly new going to them and saying I need to talk about such a thing with you, we haven't got a forum where you can do that over coffee, it has to be in the surgery and you're very conscious of that queue of people out there who've already perhaps waited a few minutes longer than they should have done and you're interrupting them to try and talk about something like this." (Ms Lacey)

The tone of Ms Lacey's opening assertion about general practitioners suggests that she does not, on the whole, consider general practitioners as approachable or particularly useful in relation to her own responsibilities as a healthcare provider. It is also pertinent that the feelings which Ms Lacey describes during her interactions with general practitioners are similar to those expressed by the participating women from stage one of this research. This is not surprising considering the relative position of women within the medical hierarchy[1], where the roles of nurses and health visitors have been assimilated into the patriarchal structure of the family generally. This suggests that the general practitioner represents the patriarchal father, other service providers such as nurses and health visitors represent the mother, and finally the patient is represented as a child (Miles, 1991; Oakley, 1993).

In relation to the interactions between nurses and doctors in particular, the distribution of power between them has historically been conceptualised within nurse/doctor game theories (Stein, 1967; Freidson, 1970) which suggest that nurses exert power through the manipulation of doctors and the maintenance of the hierarchical relationship between them. These theories have been challenged (Hughes, 1988; King et al, 1996) and it has been suggested that a negotiated order perspective (Svensson, 1996) is currently more relevant. This theory, although acknowledging the shifts in power attributable to changes within health models, for example through a shift to more holistic models of healthcare, does not recognise that the complex ways in which nurses negotiate power within the medical hierarchy could themselves represent shifts in gendered power. It could be suggested, therefore, that such theories, which challenge the traditional view of the nurse/doctor relationship within metaphors of the family structure, represent changes within that family structure rather than a deviation from it. This would be supported by arguments (Svensson, 1996) which acknowledge that, although nurses are able to negotiate more professional power in relation to their specific duties and responsibilities, they are still, ultimately, the professionals who maintain the daily care of patients beyond the physicians gaze. This role places them as mediators between the patient and the doctor/medical discourse. The negotiated order perspective, while offering explanations for the relationships between doctors and nurses, does not acknowledge that such collaborations are themselves dependent on individuals within the medical hierarchy, and within specific interactions, recognising the contribution and value of those with different professional training. It is recognised, for example, that nurse practitioners can deliver 70-80% of primary care yet are often limited from doing so (King et al, 1996). Ms Lacey clearly finds that her role places her in a contradictory position in relation to those healthcare professionals she is responsible to and her female patients.

The extracts above demonstrate that health visitors are in a particularly good position to identify domestic violence, and the health visitors who participated in this research had far more clinical experience dealing with this issue than the other second stage research participants. The impetus which this has the potential to offer the health interaction between healthcare professionals and women who experience domestic violence is lost, however, if the health visitor is prevented from taking action, in terms of advice or referrals, due to her relative position within the medical hierarchy. As has been demonstrated, this hierarchy has complex origins, particularly in relation to gender (see also Riessman, 1983; Warshaw, 1992; Candib, 1994). In relation to the responses from stage two participants, the professional relationship between health visitors and general practitioners within primary care appears to be comparable to the relationship between nurses and physicians within secondary service provision.

> "It's the younger GP in our practice to whom you can go and he'll
> be very receptive to what you're saying and it doesn't take long but
> he listens and is 'Ok, I get what you're talking about'. But certainly

the older one didn't even know what a joint medical was about ...
he's just hopeless, he's got a block where social services are concerned
and he's got certain little boxes that people go into, like she's a woman
who wants to be beaten up y'know, she's in that box, he doesn't see
that there's anything in there for him, that he could change or talk
to her about, or suggest or refer her to somewhere else.... And in
order to keep some kind of control for themselves they've got to
maintain the status quo for them haven't they, they've got to keep
the old order." (Ms Lacey)

The extract above demonstrates Ms Lacey's awareness of the medical
hierarchy and her position as a health visitor within it. While she
acknowledges the differences which exist in relation to general
practitioners as a group, she is critical of those who perpetuate the
medical hierarchy in order to maintain the position of power they hold
within the 'status quo'. This is evidence of the suggestion made earlier
that it was those medical practitioners who challenged their role as
health providers generally, and their professional and personal position
within a medical hierarchy in particular, who were more likely to consider
domestic violence, alongside other social problems, as health issues in
which they had a responsibility to intervene. The hierarchical nature of
the health service constitutes a barrier to effective collaborations between
differing healthcare providers.

Ms Lacey's comments also challenge the potential of the doctor's
role, which is conducted predominantly within the surgery and therefore
away from peoples' homes and 'real lives'. These comments demonstrate
that health visitors and practice nurses who are particularly active within
routine family healthcare are in a good position to identify, and to notify
general practitioners about, the occurrence of domestic violence, just as
they do so in relation to child protection issues. This communication
becomes difficult, however, if health visitors perceive that general
practitioners are working within a different, biomedical, health
framework.

Many of the general practitioners interviewed in stage two
acknowledged the important role which health visitors in particular
played in identifying domestic violence.

"He didn't disclose it was the health visitor who thought she
suspected, I couldn't stand the wife she was frightful, but the health
visitor suspected that the wife was violent." (Dr Eagland)

While the multi-professional approach advocated by Dr Eagland in the above extract is encouraging, it does not acknowledge the differentiation of power in the medical hierarchy. Many of the general practitioners who were interviewed suggested that if they suspected domestic violence they might ask the health visitor for her opinion and/or ask her to make a home visit. As Ms Lacey's assertions suggest, however, without the power to act on such information, the potential of the health visiting role is lost.

Counsellors

As identified in Chapter Nine, many general practitioners considered the role of the counsellor to be central in terms of the treatment options available to deal with domestic violence. This was particularly relevant to non-physical psychosomatic injuries. Appendix 1, Table A2 identifies the number of health practices in this research which had a counsellor attached to the surgery. This relationship, however, is not without its difficulties. First, counselling is a relatively new profession, in terms of in-house counselling within primary practice, and is located precariously within the medical hierarchy. This is evident in the discussions which have taken place on the evaluation and effectiveness of counselling services (House, 1996, 1997; Hudson-Allez, 1997). Humanistic counsellors (House, 1997), for example, have been critical of the way in which cost effectiveness has focused on efficiency within a biomedical model of health rather than a holistic one which would recognise the benefits of humanistic, as opposed to behavioural psychological, counselling approaches. Evaluation of the effectiveness of preventative healthcare has also been addressed, in relation to the health promotion roles of health visitors and school nurses (Billingham and Hall, 1998). It has also been suggested that, through rigid and specific accreditation procedures, the British Medical Association is recognising and promoting models of counselling within general practice which do not undermine the existing biomedical health approaches of the medical model (House, 1996). Many of these issues relate to conflicts around the professionalisation of counselling[2] within a market-driven health economy. The reality, however, is that over the past decade there has been a significant increase in the use of professional counsellors in general practice. Currently half of fundholding practices and one third of non-fundholding practices offer counselling services (Hudson-Allez, 1997; Ward and Loenenthal, 1997).

Due to the continued emergence of counselling as an important treatment option and professional resource, two counsellors were included in the second stage sample. Both counsellors, Ms Taylor and Ms Smith, referred to the existence of a 'dustbin syndrome', where they perceived general practitioners in particular as dumping any problem which they felt inadequate at dealing with onto the in-house counsellor, whether it was appropriate to make such a referral or not.

Ms Taylor discussed the approaches of three different general practitioners:

- White, middle-class man/area, who did not mention on the referral about domestic violence even though it was an issue.
- Asian GP who was over-involved and will call a perpetrator in and verbally abuse them for perpetrating the violence without concern for the effects this will have on the 'victim'.
- Third GP who repeats abusive situation by encouraging woman to stay within the violent relationship and was emotionally abusive and manipulative to the woman and the two counsellors who had both parties referred to them.

Ms Taylor's experiences of referral to her own in-house counselling service represent the diverse ways in which general practitioners respond to domestic violence and how they utilise counselling services. Ms Taylor felt she was in a position to challenge a general practitioner if his/her actions encroached on the service she provided or placed a patient at risk. Ms Taylor was employed by a number of different general practitioners, and it is questionable whether she would have felt able to challenge the views of 'her employer' had she been located within a single practice. Many of the problems concerning the referral of patients to counsellors can be located within the shifting boundaries between primary health service counsellors and secondary service provision through the community mental health team. Until the boundaries of these different roles are more clearly defined through clinical practice, there will continue to be an overlap where general practitioners are unsure about the possible benefits of each. It is acknowledged, as in Ms Taylor's assertions above, that general practitioners perceive a need for counselling support that a counsellor alone cannot meet (Ward and Loenenthal, 1997). It has also been recognised that issues of patient confidentiality can cause difficulties and barriers to effective collaboration between general practitioners and counsellors (Hudson-Allez, 1997). This problem can be compounded by the consumer model of healthcare advocated in fundholding practices, where the doctor effectively purchases the services of counsellors and thus requires confirmation of effectiveness. The issue of confidentiality and patient record-keeping was addressed in Chapter Ten.

Female general practitioners

Another issue affecting the working collaborations between healthcare professionals who are located within the medical hierarchy is the gendered differentiation within that hierarchy. All of the health visitors, practice nurses, midwives, and counsellors who took part in this research were female. This supports the view that the health professional hierarchy is based partly on the disproportionate representation of female staff in less respected, low paid occupations (Phillips and Rakusen, 1989). This differentiation was examined in the second stage interviews with general practitioners in relation to the expected roles of male and female doctors. Three of the male general practitioners stated that they perceived domestic violence to be an issue which could either be better dealt with by their female partners or which was more likely to be presented to them. Following such assertions, I subsequently asked female general practitioners to comment on this suggestion. This gendered differentiation is obviously problematic, because female general practitioners did not feel that they were more adequately positioned to treat such cases on the basis of being female. This suggests that female healthcare professionals are expected not only to deal with patients irrespective of gender, but also to treat injuries which predominantly affect women. This places women doctors within a gendered paradox in terms of professional status within a discourse which is based, arguably, on neutrality.

> "I mean that it is that which takes some more teasing out, I mean over the years because I was junior partner by a long way I used to see a lot of people like this. Now I have got two female partners I do not see as many of these cases that I used to." (Dr Fagan)

While women who experience domestic violence may wish to see female practitioners (of any profession) for the validation of their subjective experiences, the training of doctors is such that gender differentiation is reduced. In the above extract, Dr Fagan makes three assumptions. First, that domestic violence is an issue which tends to be relegated to the attention of junior doctors. Second, that female doctors are more likely to be junior doctors and therefore lower on the health professional hierarchy. Third, that female practitioners are more adequately equipped to deal with gendered issues such as domestic violence. The following extracts come from interviews with two female general practitioners:

"It's not a clear cut gender issue. On average people expect women GPs to be more approachable. One of the male partners who is particularly good at dealing with people, he has a reputation around here for being very approachable, people tend to go to him." (Dr Eagland)

[Are women GPs better at dealing with domestic violence?] "No, I wouldn't have thought so and the reason I say that is there doesn't seem to be a gendered issue in other areas. Obviously ante-natal care and gynaecology tends to be something that's brought to female doctors but we're not really talking about patients bringing in agendas, we're talking about doctors spotting something that's hidden and that's as likely to work for men and women, likely to be as bad in men and women I should think…. If it's male GPs who are saying that, what I would say to them is 'We feel just as awkward about it and just as incapacitated by it, y'know by our failure to act as they do and they shouldn't necessarily assume that we're any better at it than they are', and I would quote that evidence that there are lots of areas where gender issues are not as big an issue as the people involved think it is." (Dr Gabb)

The first extract from Dr Eagland acknowledges the perception which patients have that female general practitioners are more approachable than male doctors (Miles, 1991). She undermines this assertion, however, by claiming that the senior male partner within her surgery is well known locally for being sympathetic and approachable in relation to issues like domestic violence. Dr Gabb suggests that male and female doctors experience the same feelings of frustration in relation to issues such as domestic violence, and are likely to be equally bad at identifying such occurrences and acting on them. It is false to assume, therefore, that female doctors are more likely to provide positive interactions with women who experience domestic violence.

Primary versus secondary health services

Because the issue of communication between primary and secondary health services was raised by many of the women from stage one, I asked healthcare professionals about the 'flimsies' they received from hospitals and whether they considered the communication between themselves and secondary service providers to be adequate. This particular relationship between healthcare professionals also highlights the inconsistency of treatment of para-suicidal and crisis health intervention.

> "Well, problems with that are the accident and emergency letters are infrequent and badly written, you get very little information on them and the patient does not often report back unless they are asked to and then will tend to give whatever story they have given to A & E about it. Unless people are concerned nothing will happen. In my experience that is not the way that they presented it to me with a relatively trivial injury and then the story of domestic violence has come out. All that is presented is undeniably domestic violence was not a serious injury, ie not serious enough to go to A & E, and in those situations we will take it on from wherever it was." (Dr Fagan)

Dr Fagan denies the significance of referrals from accident and emergency departments in relation to domestic violence. This emerges out of the belief that suicide is not a significant health problem related to domestic violence, which was questioned in Chapters Three and Eight. Dr Fagan also states that the 'flimsies' general practitioners receive are often inadequate due to the way they are written and the information they contain.

> "We don't very often get those actually [flimsies]. But to start with you don't get very good communication from [the local hospital]. It may just say 'fall' or a single word 'drug-related', 'anti-inflammatory'. The [other local hospital] is better with medical reports because lists of copies of the casualty officer's actual written statement of an examination, we don't get very much at all." (Dr Habberley)

Dr Habberley identifies the variable quality of communication between primary and secondary health teams. This raises issues about the consistency of communication and documentation. It also questions the ability of different healthcare professionals to work in conjunction with one another to maximise the effectiveness of the medical interaction and health resources more generally. The historical relationship which exists between primary and secondary health providers makes the contemporary relationship between them difficult (Walker, 1988; Marshall, 1998). This problem is exacerbated by the consumer role doctors play in relation to secondary specialist services.

> "Referral letters from casualty, to answer the first bit first, are always seen by the same partner, it's his job, he gets all the flimsies from casualty and he makes an entry in all the notes and files the thing separately ... now, having said that, that's of course if we get it, and most of the discharge flimsies are given to the patient in this [geographical] area and they're brought by hand. Now you wouldn't necessarily get a record, therefore, especially if the patient is feeling sheepish about things. If you want me to identify specifically those that related to domestic violence that would have to depend on either the casualty officer (a) knew that's what the injury was caused by and (b) put it in the letter. If that did come and that was highlighted then almost certainly we would contact the patient because we do that with the para-suicides, we get the notes out of the review, who knows them best, what their circumstance are, if it's an on-going problem then that doctor will contact them. [The community psychiatric nurse] sometimes contacts new people cold so, 'I see you were in casualty last week, is there anything I can do to help?'." (Dr Gabb)

Dr Gabb's assertions above are more positive, and again we can observe an example of good practice. The fact that one member of this primary healthcare team is responsible for all the referrals from the local hospital improves the continuity of care and ensures that further interaction takes place if it is considered appropriate. This extract also suggests that other healthcare providers, in this case the community psychiatric nurse, will be informed and enlisted to assist in the appropriation of relevant healthcare. Dr Gabb also refers to the policy of giving 'flimsies' to the patient to act on. This is particularly interesting as Amy, who participated in stage one of this research, and who was a trained nurse herself, was able to avoid further health interactions following hospital treatment of both her own and her children's injuries[3] by destroying the flimsies she received. In Amy's case this was an important survival tactic in order to receive medical attention without further violence from her partner.

This raises questions about the implementation of guidelines or screening processes which remove control from the presenting patient and introduces further contradictions inherent within the medicalisation debate.

The responses of practitioners to questions about communication between local hospitals and general practices were evenly distributed between those who considered such communication to be adequate and those who were critical of the information they received. The standard of communication between local hospitals and general practices is therefore inconsistent, and is dependent on both the hospital and the medical personnel who are dealing with a particular case. Where there is a lack of recording, this results in bad communication and misdiagnoses, and creates patient records which do not adequately represent the patient's medical and/or domestic histories. This is particularly problematic for further research, as researchers who access medical records to conduct medical needs assessments in relation to domestic violence can only access partial information with which to base such assessments on (Stark and Flitcraft, 1982; Kurz, 1987; Stanko et al, 1998). Although hospitals, and accident and emergency departments in particular, may refer patients on to other specialised services, there are discrepancies as to the amount of information which gets back to the patient's general practitioner. A further issue is that there are general practices where all communication from local hospitals is followed up, and others where this is not the case. In relation to the comments made by the participating women from stage one, this lack of follow-up does not meet the needs of many women for advocacy. Many of the women felt that some kind of follow-up would represent an interest in their predicament by medical personnel but, as the above extracts demonstrate, this is not a uniform procedure. In many cases, general practice surgeries may never be made aware of the patient's attendance at the hospital accident and emergency department if the communication between the two is poor. This chapter has illustrated that there are problems inherent in the relationships between different healthcare professions. This raises concern about the ability of health practitioners to communicate adequately with other professionals whose professional ideologies may be significantly different from their own. Chapter Twelve therefore examines inter-agency collaboration beyond health services.

Notes

[1] The medical hierarchy refers to the relative position of different health professions in terms of social status, organisation, monopoly of health provision, historical emergence, training, responsibilities, and therefore power.

[2] It has been acknowledged that many general practice surgeries have always offered informal counselling, frequently provided by the wives of doctors and/or health visitors and practice nurses, see Hudson-Allez (1997).

[3] This occurred prior to the implementation of non-accidental children's registers in healthcare settings, and therefore before the 1989 Children's Act.

Wider multi-agency collaborations

From the outset this research has contextualised the health interaction between women who experience domestic violence and healthcare professionals within the wider help-seeking activities of the stage one participants. The participating women's experiences of interactions with other statutory and voluntary agencies was discussed in Chapter Five. This chapter will examine how the participating healthcare practitioners considered their interactions with other non-health professionals. In order to contextualise the qualitative extracts which will be examined below, results from the domestic violence and health questionnaire (Abbott and Williamson, 1999) found that only 14% of the respondents had been involved in multi-agency work.

Box 10: Perceptions of other agencies

The questionnaire also addressed multi-agency collaboration in relation to the responsibilities of different agencies and found that: 47.4% of respondents considered social services to have principal responsibility for domestic violence; 1.8% specifically identified health visitors; 7.3% general practitioners; 12.2% the police; 0.3% solicitors; 1.8% women's refuge; 0.5% voluntary agencies; 2.5% counsellors; and 1% mental health teams.

This chapter will begin by examining domestic violence multi-agency collaborations generally, before examining specific interactions which take place between healthcare professionals and a number of the agencies identified above.

Domestic violence multi-agency collaboration

It was identified in Chapter One that healthcare professionals have been poorly represented within domestic violence multi-agency initiatives (Hague et al, 1996). As the statistics above illustrate, only a small percentage of the participating healthcare professionals were engaged in multi-agency domestic violence work. None of the health professionals interviewed for this research were actively engaged in the local domestic violence multi-agency forum. The following extracts examine the healthcare professionals' responses to the general issue of multi-agency collaboration.

> "Obviously through the multi-disciplinary training, realising that there are other people out there too, people who struggle within their own professions with this problem, who have the same difficulties and stresses, but I think if you know faces, even vaguely, you're much happier to phone them up and say 'What should I do about, or, this is the situation I'm in where could I direct this lady?', y'know, you're much more likely to ask for help and advice if you've met somebody." (Ms Lacey)

Ms Lacey had herself benefited from domestic violence basic awareness training conducted by the local multi-agency domestic violence group. Ms Lacey identifies the importance of understanding the professional constraints which limit other professionals. She also suggests that such forums improve the communication and dissemination of information and advice between professionals on an individual and collective basis.

> "... it would be nice to have something like a register of places where you could call for help for people. Voluntary support groups right through to professional agencies." (Dr Gabb)

> "I think if I knew that there was going to be someone who was going to be sympathetic and helpful, for instance if there was, I know that the police have tried to be more sympathetic towards domestic violence, if there was a person who I knew I could contact like the police who was going to be sympathetic then I might be more, it would be helpful because if someone came to me and I thought there was a case of domestic violence then I could say if you contact so-and-so they'll be very helpful. I suppose to know where to send people I mean I ... I say very vague things like contact the police or contact social services or Citizens Advice. That sort of thing would be useful because I could give people some proper advice." (Dr Eagland)

Both Dr Gabb and Dr Eagland suggest that they require information about the other professional groups' responses and services pertaining to domestic violence. Dr Eagland refers to the need for this information in order to disseminate more appropriate information to patients who present with domestic violence-related injuries. While identifying these problems is important, because it highlights areas where the medical interaction could be improved, neither of these general practitioners is aware of the local domestic violence multi-agency action group, where different professionals meet to share information and professional experience. This organisation also holds a comprehensive county-wide resource directory relating specifically to domestic violence services. Both of these extracts also raise concerns in relation to the widely suggested treatment option of dissemination of advice and information discussed in Chapter Nine. If healthcare professionals require this basic information, which does exist, then the appropriateness of their choice of treatment options can be seriously questioned.

> "Well I do not really refer them anywhere else unless you know that there is a serious psychiatric problem or something like that like depression, you know which I might treat myself, or if it is too severe refer to the psychiatric clinic." (Dr Iannelli)

Dr Iannelli locates his professional role in relation to a narrowly defined medical interaction which precludes the possibility of dealing adequately with a number of health problems which have social origins. His suggestion that he would himself treat minor psychological symptoms without considering alternative resources illustrates how the medical profession has become isolated from other professional practice.

> "I think that the social back-up is generally very good and liaison is very good with them concerned about people, you know the liaison from probation services, from the police, from the psychiatric services, these are very helpful. Where you have other major problems, where you just deal with domestic violence, there is not a lot of help because if you are geared to deal with people with criminal records, with people with alcohol and drugs problems, with people with HIV-related problems, again the focus is on those things and not on the violence issue. So violence is an area which does not receive a great deal of priority as far as I can see." (Dr Fagan)

Dr Fagan identifies the difficulties and frustrations which arise when a number of social issues exist in conjunction with domestic violence. Rather than compounding these frustrations, however, multi-agency collaboration can assist professionals in dealing with a multitude of issues simultaneously. Most notably, through the appropriate use of specific services which acknowledge domestic violence in conjunction with these other problems[1]. In relation to Dr Fagan's comments, it is important to note that the local domestic violence multi-agency forum has representatives from a diverse range of agencies. These include those who focus on alcohol and drug dependency, voluntary health support groups, and disability focus groups among others. While these professionals, statutory or otherwise, have a specific focus within their own work, they still acknowledge the importance of domestic violence, both in relation to that work and independently.

The assertions made in the above extracts are positive, on the whole, as they identify the contribution that multi-agency initiatives can have on the working environment. The problems which have been identified, such as a register of local statutory and voluntary services, and also being able to contact an individual rather than a 'faceless' agency, are problems the answers to which already exist locally (within a 20-mile radius) for all the healthcare professionals who were interviewed for this research. The local domestic violence multi-agency initiative, which is fortunate to currently employ two people[2], one a project coordinator, holds a directory of all the service provision available to women experiencing domestic violence throughout the county. They also coordinate various multi-agency forums where a diverse range of professionals meet to discuss problems and issues relating to domestic violence within their own workloads. As stated at the outset of this book, this research is concerned with the medical professions' response to domestic violence, partly because their lack of representation within multi-agency domestic violence forums has become problematic for women experiencing violence, and for other professional groups whose involvement has led to the development and implementation of better services and safeguards to service provision. The lack of knowledge which healthcare professionals have about domestic violence is directly related to this lack of representation in these multi-agency collaborations. It is not surprising, however, that the majority of the participating healthcare professionals, and general practitioners in particular, focused on the inadequacies of others rather than their own lack of active participation in existing support networks.

> "Because it can't be anybody else in the first instance because we are the first point of call. If people come in with an injury you've got to deal with. It's all very well saying it's a problem for social services or it's a problem for the church or a problem for schools, but everybody has to be involved and we're just one agency." (Dr Gabb)

This assertion is crucial as it rightly identifies the need to acknowledge that women access healthcare services for advice, treatment and support for specific reasons. Although using multi-agency networks for professional support, information, and in order to assist referral procedures is positive, healthcare professionals need to acknowledge that if a woman wished to contact the police or social services it is likely she would do so as part of her own wider help-seeking activities. Women utilise healthcare services because they require treatment for physical and non-physical injuries and because health services are confidential and accessible. Is is imperative, therefore, that healthcare professionals take seriously their collaborative role with other statutory and voluntary service providers in order to maximise their skills and resources. Only by doing so will they ensure that they too offer women a range of options with which to negotiate violent and abusive relationships.

The police

The police[3] and the legal system more generally have already been mentioned by the second stage participants as an important resource for women experiencing domestic violence. Even within general definitions of domestic violence (see Chapter Six), a number of participating healthcare professionals referred to the legal implications of domestic violence as a crime. Stage one participants too referred to the ways in which the police were accessed as a source of help within an abusive situation. How the participating health professionals perceived the police in relation to domestic violence is therefore important in a multi-agency context.

> "The biggest tricky bit is when you get people who walk in like I said earlier and say 'Well the police has asked me to come for a report', and I find that difficult. I'd rather if the police officer was going to do that that somebody from the domestic violence unit wrote and said 'Mrs so-and-so has presented and can you tell us...' and ask for a report that's explicit. I find it difficult when they just walk in off the street and you have to start making notes." (Dr Gabb)

The above quotation specifically requests greater collaboration with the police in relation to domestic violence cases. Unfortunately, while this extract is encouraging in that it identifies a specific way in which multi-agency collaboration could be initiated, the police are already represented on many of the multi-agency forums. Indeed, many domestic violence multi-agency initiatives were begun with collaboration and backing from the police. The above extract may, therefore, say more about the lack of representation of healthcare professionals within those initiatives rather than a lack of communication from the police themselves.

> "I often don't know what they come for. Because at the end of the day all you can really say, we haven't really got any powers to stop this happening, all we can really say is 'Look I think you should go to the police and get an injunction taken out for your own safety and for the safety of your kids'. I think they just want to come and open up and tell somebody, just to get it off their chests." (Dr Padden)

While the above extract demonstrates an awareness that domestic violence is a legally defined crime, in light of the experiences of the stage one participants, professionals need to be aware of the effects of seeking professional help, and the barriers which prevent women from prosecuting, leaving or challenging their abusive partners' behaviour.

The help-seeking experiences of the stage one participants in relation to the police were examined in Chapter Five. The participating women often felt frustrated by the inadequate response of the police, and their preoccupation with obtaining statements. Healthcare professionals need to be aware, therefore, that women access professionals for a variety of reasons, and may access health services for specific help and assistance which cannot be offered by other professionals at that time.

Social services

The non-medical professionals most frequently cited in the second stage interviews were social services. While social services may be an important resource where children are present in a domestically violent situation, their appropriateness outside of this context is questionable. The following extracts demonstrate a range of perceptions and experiences of healthcare professionals' multi-agency collaboration with social services.

> "I think they're happy to refer, I think we're all now happy to refer in many ways, we don't think sort of think we're omnipotent, we know there are lots of other services available and I think we have a better communication between our services. I think the health visitors they link up with social services very quickly and again with GPs if

there's obvious physical abuse, but when we're talking about mental
abuse that's a very different thing, how can you refer anyone to
anyone really, I mean where is the answer?" (Ms Naylor)

Ms Naylor is competent at using multi-agency networks due to her
role as a health visitor and the responsibility she has to interact with
other professionals in relation to child protection issues. None of the
health visitors who were interviewed for this research had a problem in
relation to multi-agency collaboration. Ms Naylor's assumption that
her colleagues have as much knowledge and information about other
service providers as she does is misplaced, however, as the earlier extracts
concerning an acknowledged lack of information demonstrated.

"There's no defined role or no defined position as to where the
boundaries between NHS and social workers should be. The higher
up managerially-wise the more they're trying to pass it over to the
other side. At ground level it usually becomes a scrap as to everybody
I think, trying to do their best but not having the resources to help,
it usually ends up being passed down the line until it's somewhere
where there's nobody else to pass it to and they do the donkey work.
You asked about health visitors, GPs are as guilty as anyone else of
passing it on if someone comes into the surgery in tears and says
their husband's been emotionally and verbally abusive to them and
we might ask the health visitor to see what we can do, or refer on to
the charities or whatever else. The people I've not used very much
because I think clients/patients are reluctant to see is the police who
I believe have a domestic violence unit, but there's a real barrier to
people going to the police, especially in communities where they
tend to be poorer and I think the only contact people have had with
the police has tended to be very negative in the past, they've been
arrested for this, that and the other or they know someone who has.
There's still resentment from the miners' strike from 10 years ago
around here and I think to some extent despite what the police try
and do they're always seen as the enemy, which is why they come to
the doctor because we're apolitical and non-judgmental as much as
we can be.... I think social workers have got a place but again social
workers have got a bit of a bad reputation as well, seen as the people
who come and take your kids away, I think if you get onto the social
workers' books it looks very bad, or that's how the patients see it.
Which I think is where general practitioners and the health service
tends to bear the brunt of it. I think people do know there is

confidentiality, there is still respect for GPs that you will try and do whatever you can, it's just we can't keep up with their respective issues." (Dr Padden)

I have included this lengthy extract from the interview with Dr Padden as it contains a number of significant points relating to multi-agency collaboration. First, he acknowledges the power inherent in the relationship between doctors and health visitors, and suggests that general practitioners frequently 'pass the buck'. This validates the extracts from health visitors discussed earlier. Second, Dr Padden refers to professional boundaries between social and medical services. This relates specifically to medicalised problems, where the jurisdiction between the two professional groups becomes increasingly blurred.

"Again, much as there's trouble between various patients, social services and GPs are just at each others' throats, there's this pure confrontational relationship. The only time I speak to social services is when I ring up and say I've just had Mr Bloggs go into hospital, his wife is at home on her own and she needs looking after. It's just pure out and out confrontation all round, or if they go round and they've had home help, in they can no longer get Mrs Bloggs out of bed, they just dump it on us and say ... our relationship is just terrible." (Dr Padden)

Expanding on the relationship between social services and healthcare professionals which Dr Padden referred to previously, he suggests that the relationship between the two is based on confrontation. The shifting boundaries which appear to be responsible for this conflict support the idea that there exists a so-called 'health crisis' as a result of increased medicalisation, and that healthcare professionals are finding it increasingly difficult to address the problems they are presented with within a medical framework. Hence the assertion that in many cases it is the responsibility of social services to deal with particular problems. This relates directly to the relationship between professionalism and the process of medicalisation discussed earlier (Chapter Eleven), in the context of the existence of gendered power relations within the medical hierarchy.

"I honestly wouldn't be able to tell you where the nearest refuge is. I would ring up, if I'd got a situation, y'know if a crisis had developed and I was worried about somebody's physical and mental health and I thought they needed emergency care I'd ring social services' duty officer, who is always available, not always helpful ... at the end of the day I have always got facilities through the NHS for a bed overnight but that's not an answer by any means." (Dr Padden)

This extract identifies the emergency resources which healthcare professionals have at their disposal, and it was the only reference made in the second stage interviews to the possibility of giving a woman a bed overnight in order to escape a domestically violent situation. Dr Padden also admits that he does not have information about domestic violence refuges and would again rely on social services for this information. This lack of knowledge and subsequent reliance on social services could itself be partly responsible for the conflictual relationship Dr Padden suggests exists between the providers of both social services and healthcare.

> "I suppose a sort of quicker assessment of a situation, more, it's difficult isn't it, sort of ... I mean trying to sort of network with social workers and people to sort of get a common ... and I think [we] have actually got a good relationship with social services, I've had sort of pre-meetings, social workers have phoned up and said 'I'm just about to go and what's your angle on it and we've had a sort of quick network meeting on it', when that works it works really well, when it doesn't work then you end up with numerous agencies working in different directions and saying well ... and you're relying on the patient almost for Chinese whispers, it gets distorted and...."
> (Dr Jabber)

The comments made in the above extracts vary in the experiences healthcare professionals have had with social services, and whether they perceive that interaction as positive or not. Clearly, healthcare professionals see social services not only as a service provider in themselves, but also as responsible for referral to other agencies. While the duty social worker may have such information, it must be extremely frustrating to have to deal with such cases when the healthcare professional is just as capable of referring to appropriate agencies directly. Another issue is the way in which healthcare professionals believe the presenting women, and the community at large, to perceive other agencies. If healthcare professionals believe that women will not access social services and the police, for whatever reason, it makes more sense to contact the appropriate services directly. Where collaboration has occurred, as in the experiences of Dr Jabber and Ms Naylor, this experience has resulted in a better service and has provided the healthcare professional with vital information and the professional support of others. Multi-agency collaborations would assist in widening the support networks currently available to healthcare professionals. They would also enable healthcare providers to take advantage of their professional position within society as a confidential statutory service provider which does not, on the whole, have the same social stigma as do agencies such as social services and the police.

Voluntary agencies

So far I have focused specifically on extracts which refer to statutory agencies. The following extracts refer to the multi-agency collaboration which occurs between healthcare professionals and voluntary service providers. As mentioned earlier in relation to the results of the domestic violence and health questionnaire (Abbott and Williamson, 1999), just over 2% of respondents considered voluntary agencies (including women's refuges) to have responsibility for dealing with domestic violence. Respondents also stated that they would like more information about locally available services and provision. Bearing these responses in mind, it was not surprising that the majority of stage two participants had little or inadequate knowledge about voluntary services.

> "Well quite honestly no. I do not feel that there is anything much at all locally and the sort of hostels for women who are victims of violence are a long way away. The decision to go to such hostels mean how do they get there and takes them away from their family support and it means disrupting the children and these sort of situations prevent people from seeking advice. I do not feel adequately informed because the last thing that I had about women from the … Centre in [the city] and there was a set-up for women in violence and that seems to have disappeared or at least I tried to find it recently and could not get it. The only thing that I could get was the [telephone] line and that was not really appropriate." (Dr Fagan)

> "We sometimes refer them to the women's centre … for further counselling and advice." (Dr Iannelli)

There is clearly a need for more widespread dissemination of information about voluntary sector services which cater for the needs of women experiencing domestic violence, both directly and indirectly. Knowing the existence of a specific long-term and well established voluntary service, as in both extracts included above, does not represent an adequate knowledge of local voluntary service provision, particularly when such services are often underfunded or only funded for short periods of time. As mentioned earlier, an up-to-date resource directory exists for such services, but is clearly not being utilised by healthcare professionals either as an alternative, or in addition to, multi-agency domestic violence forums. Healthcare professionals need to be aware of the existence of these services so that they can access information, services and support. There is also a problem with the provision of services being less accessible to those women living in rural and isolated areas. This is not a criticism of the voluntary sector, as they are constantly underfunded and dependent on short-term funding allocations for their survival, but it is a very real problem, which Dr Fagan rightly identifies above.

Considering the frustrations caused by lack of resources, and this was by far the most acknowledged barrier to effective clinical practice, the lack of information which the stage two participants had in relation to additional voluntary services is alarming. While such services are frequently underfunded, a number of voluntary sector organisations exist, both nationally and locally, to provide services specifically for women experiencing domestic violence. Because the participating healthcare professionals have little knowledge about these services they are again experiencing frustrations within their clinical practice rather than maximising their own potential. This will be addressed in relation to the recommendations of this book in Chapter Fourteen. This chapter has examined inter-agency collaboration in relation to domestic violence. There are wider issues for health providers, relating to the way in which health practitioners interact with other professionals more generally. These issues relate directly to the ways in which health practitioners are trained, as well as to the epistemologies adopted within medical and non-medical education. Chapter Thirteen addresses the issue of training, both generally and in relation to domestic violence.

Notes

[1] For example, the Leeds Domestic Violence Multi-agency Project has successfully monitored the repeat victimisation perpetrated by abusers and has subsequently been able to identify where specific services (such as drug rehabilitation services) are required to combat the crime of domestic violence.

[2] Since this book has been re-edited, the local multi-agency group has lost its funding and no longer employs a coordinator. It is still important to

acknowledge, however, that throughout the four-and-a-half years when this research was being conducted a coordinator was employed specifically to liaise with a range of statutory and voluntary agencies. As in other areas of the country, healthcare professionals were under-represented.

[3] For specific information concerning police multi-agency initiatives, see Hanmer et al (1999), Kelly (1999), Bridgeman and Hobbs (1997) and Plotnikoff and Woolfson (1998).

THIRTEEN

Training

All the professional relationships examined in the previous two chapters have inherent within them an element of conflict based on the different professional ideologies of practitioners, both within and beyond the health professions. The reasons why communication is particularly poor in some instances are related directly to the way in which those in positions of authority, for example the general practitioner, perceive their role in society, and how they negotiate the power which is afforded that position. If a general practitioner perceives their own role in relation to the other services offered by their less respected (and paid) colleagues, then collaboration with those individuals is likely to be more productive. This is evident in new training approaches, which are attempting to implement changes in undergraduate medical training, from a biomedical/wound-led hospital approach to one which is community based and holistically located. The issue of training, considering the importance of training in relation to the acquisition of professional status, is paramount in offering health practitioners knowledge with which to inform their clinical practice. Training, in content and methodology, is also important for teaching new professionals their responsibilities, particularly in relation to the roles of others. In light of these considerations, this chapter will begin by examining medical training generally, before considering the concept of community-based and holistic training methods. Returning to the specific issue of domestic violence, this chapter will also address the impact of multi-agency training, before examining the concept of specialised training on domestic violence for healthcare professionals.

Community-based training models

It has been suggested that the modern healthcare system is currently in a state of crisis (Davis, 1979; Stark, 1982; Lowenberg and Davis, 1994), where the costs of providing adequate healthcare outweigh the funding available for such services. In documenting this 'crisis' in health provision, medical sociologists have examined how the role of the medic and the social control function of the medical profession are having to change to withstand these developments, while simultaneously maintaining the status of the profession. The historical origins of the medical profession suggest that the current 'health crisis' is due to the inability of medical discourse to treat adequately many of the medicalised problems which came under its jurisdiction in the process of professionalisation (Turner, 1995). Medical training, too, has specific historical origins beyond the philosophical paradigmatic shifts which facilitated the emergence of medical discourse[1]. Despite the incorporation in early medical training of psychosocial factors beyond the physician's 'gaze' (Lyons and Petrucelli, 1987), the emergence of teaching hospitals resulted in training which was clinically focused in relation to procedures and treatments within a biomedical model of healthcare (Flexner, 1912; Osler, 1951). The shift away from this paradigm is evident in moves towards community education as one way in which to produce medics able to deal more adequately with public health problems in their widest sense. Whitehouse et al (1997) have examined the advantages of community-based medical training and suggest that:

> The community provides access to a more 'normal' sector of society, to more common and more long-term health problems, to prevention and public health. Within the community it is much easier to obtain a holistic overview of patients and their health needs. Problems can be seen from the time they first present to the doctor until final resolution by recovery or death; problems can be seen within the psychosocial and environmental contexts; problems can be seen from the perspectives of all the participants – health professionals and carers alike. (Whitehouse et al, 1997, pp 16-17)

The above quotation outlines the advantages of community-based learning by suggesting that it provides a more holistic concept of healthcare. Whitehouse et al also suggest that community-based learning enables teachers to utilise problem-based learning methodologies, which produces health professionals who are able to continue to learn beyond their initial medical training without the overload of information which is particularly problematic for medical students. Indeed, the community-based learning methods suggested above are also highly conducive to the aims of the General Medical Council itself (GMC, 1993). Through a series of objectives which focus on more holistic, community-based medical training, the GMC suggests that the overall aim of medical education is to "produce a caring doctor competent to deliver the highest quality of healthcare, able to advance the science of medicine and eager to go on learning more" (Whitehouse et al, 1997, p 30). Defining the type of medic that professional bodies wish to see being produced as a result of intensive training is particularly important in relation to the need within community-based primary practice to work alongside other professional groups.

> ... there is a risk that medical students, having been high achievers at school, and succeeding in a course that is certainly intellectually challenging, might hold the view that they, as part of the medical profession, are (almost) omniscient and omnipotent. This is not a helpful attitude, as it predisposes to arrogance, and leads to despair when the truth eventually dawns! Students should acquire awareness of their personal limitations, and of the need to seek help when necessary (GMC Objectives 3 (h)). This will include seeking help from other team members and requires the development of team-working skills and exploring attitudes to other health professionals. (Whitehouse et al, 1997, p 50)

As the quotation above acknowledges, learning about how to work as a member of a team is a skill which medical practitioners need to acquire. As has been demonstrated by comments from other health practitioners in previous chapters, it is also a skill which would be appreciated by many other health professionals working in primary practice.

Research which has evaluated community-based medical training (Lennox and Petersen, 1998) suggests that students taught in an inter-agency environment will integrate better into multi-disciplinary health teams. In such research, students reported having a better awareness of psychosocial factors affecting health and were more open to holistic and inter-agency health approaches (Lennox and Petersen, 1998). Just as this example demonstrates that the training and education of healthcare professionals are having to adjust to take account of community-based inter-agency models of healthcare, so too the government's acknowledgement of inter-agency collaborations generally should influence further developments in this direction (Griffiths, 1998).

The multi-agency collaborations discussed in Chapter Twelve in relation to domestic violence do not exist in a health vacuum. The current trend in medical education is towards more community-based training, around issues which facilitate problem-based learning and greater inter-agency collaboration. Domestic violence is exactly such an issue, requiring a problem-based approach within an holistic inter-agency context. Domestic violence, as has been demonstrated throughout this book, has inherent within it a number of contradictions relating to the family, law, medicine, subjectivity, gender, and cultural discourses. As such, domestic violence would be an ideal area on which to focus community-based medical training. This will be outlined further in Chapter Fourteen, in relation to the recommendations of this text; however, any moves towards community-based professional health training and methods of working must be encouraged and supported. As this book has demonstrated, working in isolation is producing significant frustrations for health professionals which are acting as barriers to 'good practice' in relation to the experiences of women who present with domestic violence-related injuries.

Training healthcare professionals about domestic violence

A number of problems have emerged throughout this book relating to the way in which healthcare professionals interact with patients who have experienced domestic violence. A number of stage two participants acknowledged that they lack information about domestic violence services, as well as issues about domestic violence more generally. This is not surprising, considering that 86% of respondents to the domestic violence and health questionnaire (Abbott and Williamson, 1999) stated that they had inadequate knowledge about domestic violence. A further 89.3% said that they had not addressed the issue of domestic violence as part of their basic medical/health training, and only 11.1% had done so in postgraduate training. It was also interesting that a student nurse present as an observer at one of the interviews had not addressed the issue of domestic violence and did not believe that it was part of her curriculum.

The results obtained from the domestic violence and health questionnaire, as well as the qualitative data included in this book, are supported by literature from North America. Parsons et al (1995) found that, from a sample of obstetricians and gynaecologists who completed a domestic violence questionnaire, 313 (33.9%) indicated that they had no education in domestic violence. In addition, 429 (48.9%) agreed or strongly agreed that they felt inadequate in dealing with abuse because of a lack of training. Furthermore, and particularly important in relation to screening, 'lack of education and training including the difficulty in dealing with psychosocial issues' was the most common potential barrier to screening (71% of respondents identified this as a problematic area for health professionals) (Parsons et al, 1995).

The lack of training which healthcare professionals receive about domestic violence is alarming, and has been acknowledged by some healthcare professionals (Friend et al, 1998) and researchers (Hague et al, 1996) in Britain. Although the generic training currently offered to professionals in Britain has been acknowledged and praised (Friend et al, 1998, p 320), very little is known about specific programmes of training developed for healthcare professionals[2]. One study examined the effectiveness of a domestic violence course focused on a pilot domestic violence training module which was taught to undergraduate medical students (Schoonmaker and Shull, 1994). This domestic violence module consisted of two four-hour sessions which centred around an interview between a clinician and a 'standardised patient' who was trained as a domestic violence victim (standardised patients are often used within radical training to enable student interactions with patients to be evaluated in a uniform manner). The undergraduate students taking this programme were also asked to take a pre-test which was designed to measure their initial baseline knowledge of the subject area. Following the interview, students received a presentation which included sections on definitions, recognition of signs and symptoms, legal issues, and interviewing techniques. Students were then split into smaller groups where they were given the opportunity to engage with standardised patients themselves, before a final presentation addressing the limits of the caregiver's responsibility, the barriers physicians must acknowledge, and the role of other agencies. Students were finally asked to complete a post-test which was compared with their previous responses. The authors clearly acknowledge a number of problems associated with the use of standardised patients, not least that they "learned early on that training and debriefing these standardised patients are more time consuming than they are in cases with less complicated subject matter" (Schoonmaker and Shull, 1994, p 412). While being able to empathise with a woman who has experienced domestic violence is important, utilising standardised patients is problematic, as it suggests that standardised domestic violence patients exist[3]. Empathy is an important element of training, however, which has been addressed elsewhere, for example through students studying books (fiction and non-fiction) which illustrate individual feelings about domestic violence (Campbell, 1992). Schoonmaker and Shull (1994) also encountered problems relating to students' confusion of the pre- and post-test questionnaires. Having acknowledged these problems, however, the authors state that students found the subject of considerable interest and were keen to engage with standardised patients.

Training healthcare professionals about their roles in relation to domestic violence is a complex issue. First, the diversity of health professions, and the hierarchical structure within which it is maintained, influence the ways in which different health professionals are trained, as well as how they are able to practice healthcare. Second, the amount of social issues which have undergone medicalisation is already influencing and contributing to the intensity of existing training. Finally, it has been suggested that medical training is based on principles which themselves mirror abusive relationships (Warshaw, 1992). Despite these problems (and in relation to the third point, maybe because of them), domestic violence is, as has been illustrated throughout this book, a very serious, time-consuming, frustrating public health issue which healthcare professionals are being asked to deal with. Training is central to any recommendations which attempt to improve interactions between healthcare professionals and patients who present with domestic violence-related injuries. Considering the complexity of domestic violence, it is important that domestic violence training addresses not only the medical and health effects of domestic violence but, as this research has done, contextualises that knowledge within the social, cultural and professional discourses which impact on the experience of domestic violence. Literature which examines training for health professionals predominantly offers an holistic model which encompasses these different perspectives. For example, Hadley (1992) suggests that training topics should include: education on domestic violence; the effects of violence on children; resources; medical system recognition and response; and volunteer and programme procedures (Hadley, 1992, p 21). In relation to components focusing specifically on domestic violence, Hadley includes sections on: definitions; statistics; myths and realities; dynamics of abuse; cycle of violence; responsibility of behaviour; challenging the questions, "why she stays?" / "why does he do it?"; mental health issues; sexual abuse and assault; chemical use, abuse and dependency; legal advocacy; and working with men who batter. Beginning any domestic violence and health training with a substantial component addressing the realities of domestic violence and challenging the cultural myths which pervade society is warranted, not least by the data illustrated in the results and analysis chapters of this book. Hadley also includes training components which encourage health professionals to consider their medical responsibilities in relation to policy and practice.

Training has also been used in a number of initiatives to increase the identification of domestic violence cases (Stark and Flitcraft, 1996), as well as to improve the services women who experience domestic violence receive (Campbell, 1992)[4]. Domestic violence training, which is often creative and imaginative in its approach, has also been credited with helping to reshape pedagogical concepts within medical training itself (Campbell, 1992). There are, therefore, a number of positive contributions which the inclusion of domestic violence on health curricula would facilitate. Despite the relative slowness of the health professions generally to respond to the British government's calls, in 1995, to engage in the inter-agency process, it is hoped that such moves may yet occur.

Domestic violence training tools

The following sections introduce a range of training tools which could be used to facilitate domestic violence training. Such training should be conducted in consultation with women's advocates, in order to ensure that it addresses the issue of domestic violence adequately and sensitively. The following examples are included in order to illustrate how very clear and concise exercises can begin to undermine stereotypical preconceived ideas about domestic violence patients, and to reduce the many frustrations which the second stage participants in this research identified. In all of the following examples, it should be remembered that women may not be able to take leaflets or other information away with them, due to reprisals from perpetrators of domestic violence. This should not, however, prevent health practitioners from discussing the issue of domestic violence and, in particular, issues of safety with patients. Research has demonstrated (Easteal, 1994; Glass, 1995) that women remember good advice and sensitive professionals, and often utilise the advice at a later date in order to survive.

Medical power and control wheel

Schornstein (1997) addresses the issue of domestic violence and health, and includes within that consideration a number of issues specifically relevant to training. In particular, Schornstein uses a 'medical power and control wheel' and an 'advocacy wheel' (Cosgrove, 1992) in order to illustrate how healthcare professionals' practice can be either part of the problems experienced by women experiencing domestic violence or, alternatively, part of the solution[5]. The medical power and control wheel identifies a number of negative medical interventions which in themselves contribute to escalating danger and increased entrapment for the domestic violence patient. The following points are addressed on each wheel, once through identifying negative professional practice, and a second time contextualised with examples of 'good practice' (Schornstein, 1997).

- The wheel identifies how practitioners can violate confidentiality by interviewing the woman in front of her family, by discussing issues with other colleagues without the patient's consent, and by contacting the police or other agencies without the patient's consent.
- Practitioners may trivialise and minimise the abuse by not taking the danger the woman perceives seriously or by expecting tolerance due to the number of years the woman may already have spent within the relationship.
- Normalising victimisation through failing to respond to disclosures of domestic violence, either because of the acceptance that intimidation in relationships is normal, or that violence is the outcome of non-compliance with patriarchy.
- Practitioners can also exacerbate the problem of domestic violence by failing to acknowledge the woman's need for safety. This is compounded when the practitioner may be unwilling to ask the woman whether it is actually safe to return home, or whether the woman has somewhere else to go if the violence escalates.
- Blaming the victim is identified through the questions practitioners may ask, such as asking what the patient did to provoke an incident of abuse, or by focusing on her as the problem, challenging why she doesn't leave, or by asking the patient why she lets her partner treat her abusively.
- Finally, the medical power and control wheel identifies how not respecting the patient's autonomy through 'prescribing' solutions and punishing her when she does not take such advice, also contributes to the way in which medical intervention can itself be part of the problem.

This particular model offers solutions in relation to: respecting the patient's confidentiality; believing and validating her experiences; acknowledging the injustice of abuse; helping the patient to plan for future safety; promoting access to community services; and respecting her autonomy. This type of advocacy attempts to address many of the problems which have emerged as significant in this book. It identifies how specific actions can either help or hinder a domestic violence patient. As a training tool, the medical power and control wheel has a visual impact which, rather than being linear, addresses a series of important issues holistically. This adds to a focus on holistic/person-led medical approaches.

Interviewing strategies

The issue of screening has been introduced at various points in this text. Integrally linked to the concept of screening is communication. The reluctance of healthcare professionals to ask their patients about domestic violence was discussed in Chapters Nine and Ten, in relation to different treatment options and documentation. Failing to ask about the origins of a domestic violence-related injury not only makes diagnosis difficult, but precludes the possibility of healthcare professionals offering sympathetic advice and support to women who have been abused. As a result of this reluctance, a number of health professionals and domestic violence advocates (Sheridan, 1993; Varvaro and Lasko, 1993; Chez, 1994; Butler, 1995; Denham, 1995; Norton et al, 1995) have developed lists of questions intended to make healthcare professionals feel more comfortable about how to approach the subject of domestic violence with their patients. The way in which these questions are worded is intended to enable healthcare professionals to feel comfortable approaching the subject of domestic violence while also being supportive of their patients and creating an environment conducive to disclosure. Such lists frequently include questions relating to observations which the healthcare professional may have made, for example, "I noticed you have a number of bruises. Could you tell me how that happened? Did someone hit you?" (Schornstein, 1997, p 76). They also encourage healthcare professionals to support the patient by informing her that they themselves are not shocked, and that domestic violence is a common and important part of their work. For example, by telling the woman "we see many women in the ED (emergency department) with injuries like the one(s) you have. Can you tell me how the injury happened?" (Varvaro and Lasko, 1993, p 40). Other questions can address issues of safety, by ensuring that the patient is not minimising the danger she is in. Finally, scripted questions can be worded to offer patients validation of their experiences while being simultaneously conducive to disclosure.

Such assessment devices and screening tools are intended to enable the healthcare professional to obtain sensitive information within an empowering framework. Research which has examined the effectiveness of such tools has found that women are three times more likely to report experiences of domestic violence when asked specific questions from abuse assessment devices than through routine interviews (Norton et al, 1995, p 323). This same research found that more women (29%) admitted having experienced abuse when questioned by a health provider, compared to women who were asked to fill out an assessment form themselves (8%). This has implications for research, as well as for the education and training of healthcare professionals. As both a clinical and training tool, this method enables students to examine their own cultural misconceptions and apprehensions about domestic violence within a problem-based learning environment.

Female injury location chart

The issue of documentation was addressed in depth in Chapter Ten. In conjunction with problems arising from disclosure there were also discrepancies in relation to note taking and documentation. The female injury location chart (Schornstein, 1997) is one example of a visual teaching aid which can be used within training to stress the importance of documenting domestic violence-related physical injuries accurately. This clinical resource is both quick to utilise and, if used properly, would enable the clinician to provide forensic notes within a limited time period. Such visual aids would assist future practitioners in quickly identifying repeat injuries and the potential risk of long-term health implications. This would consequently give the practitioner more time in consultations to talk to patients about issues of safety, offer advice and information, and validate patients' non-physical injuries.

Danger assessment and safety planning

One of the first and most important things a healthcare professional can do for a woman experiencing domestic violence is to assess her danger and to devise a safety plan. As has already been illustrated, this should not be used as a way in which to coerce a woman to leave a violent partner, although stating that you are genuinely concerned for a patient may help to make them feel valued and therefore assist them in making positive and healthy choices despite the existence of violence and abuse.

The information card safety plan (Schornstein, 1997) is one method of raising the issue of safety with a woman experiencing domestic violence. It includes suggestions which a woman may need to take into account in order to improve her safety. These suggestions include: breaking the silence about violence by telling a friend or family member; planning for an escape by thinking about all possible escape routes in the event of an attack; planning a safe place to go once you have left;

leaving important documents such as birth certificates, benefits books, passports, and keys with someone you can trust; trying to save some money in your own name; having letters sent to a friend's address; knowing your rights; and finally suggesting that if you are in danger, do not wait – call the emergency services.

Information can also be disseminated in the form of a statement of rights (Schornstein, 1997), which is a brief summary of a woman's legal and social rights if she has experienced domestic violence. This includes outlining the types of information a woman should expect from a range of professionals, as well as the financial cost of specific services. Finally, Schornstein (1997) identifies a standardised danger assessment instrument which asks questions which can assist practitioners in assessing the potential risk a woman experiencing domestic violence is in. As mentioned earlier, this tool can be useful in helping a woman to acknowledge the danger of a situation she may have learned to minimise; it should not, however, be used to coerce a patient or remove her choices and thus her control of the consultation.

All of these tools can be used by trainers to highlight lack of knowledge and teach healthcare professionals about the services which a patient can expect to access within the locality, as well as offering clinical resources which can be used by health practitioners to work positively with women experiencing domestic violence.

Standardised patients

The concept of standardised patients was mentioned earlier in relation to research which has examined the effectiveness of domestic violence and health training (Schoonmaker and Shull, 1994). These researchers acknowledged the limitations of this training method, specifically in relation to resources; however, the role of "patients as partners in medical education" (Kelly, 1997, p 27) has been acknowledged as an important training resource, particularly in relation to community-based training methods. Both St Bartholomew's Hospital and the Royal London Hospital School of Medicine have adopted 'patients as partners' as a learning approach (Kelly, 1997). While using women who have experienced domestic violence in training would require careful monitoring, preferably by a women's organisation such as Women's Aid, 'survivor's' perspectives are already included in many inter-agency basic awareness training courses. The representation of women who have experienced domestic violence as 'experts' within training can also facilitate the identification of both good and bad practice.

The dangers of this approach, however, should also be acknowledged, and until healthcare professionals demonstrate their willingness to move beyond a biomedical approach to healthcare, such training methods may not prove effective or ethical. As an alternative, asking students to locate themselves as standardised patients by learning about domestic violence from the available literature would be a viable alternative. Campbell (1992), for example, began a domestic violence training course with nurses by requiring them to read a number of semi-fictional books which addressed violence and abuse from the 'victim's' perspective. Used in conjunction with material which has identified a number of case studies from existing professional files (Stanko et al, 1998), this approach can teach students about the experience of domestic violence without the risks of employing standardised patients.

Screening

The reluctance of the participating healthcare professionals to ask patients about domestic violence, even when presented with identified domestic violence-related injuries, has effectively undermined any serious consideration of screening for domestic violence as a matter of routine. Screening and documentation, however, are integrally linked, and in order to contribute to the more holistic training methods which have been suggested (Whitehouse et al, 1997), screening is included here as a training tool. Addressing screening has implications, not only for individual patients and practices, but for the teaching of public health more generally. Lazzaro and McFarlane (1991) suggest a number of steps which are necessary in order to establish an effective screening programme for abused women. These steps include:

• Establishing effective documentation.
• Obtaining broad-based agency support.
• Identifying common resources.
• Identifying key personnel.
• Providing staff education.
• Updating community resources.
• Providing staff support.

Again, as with the other suggestions illustrated here, this approach incorporates the key elements of any domestic violence and health training which includes an inter-agency approach, examining the wider experience of domestic violence, as well as the help-seeking context within which the health interaction takes place. Asking students to consider the implementation of domestic violence screening highlights the lack of information and documentation which currently exists; it requires students to think about the structure of healthcare in a reflexive manner and, if taught within a problem-based framework, would enable students to consider the current prevalence of domestic violence as an issue facing a range of professional agencies both nationally and internationally.

This chapter has examined shifts in medical training and introduced a number of training tools which, it has been suggested, would be useful in developing domestic violence and health training for a range of healthcare professionals. These tools are versatile in their multi-agency focus and offer medical trainers the opportunity to advance the community- and problem-based learning approaches which have been adopted to take the medical curriculum into the twenty-first century (Whitehouse et al, 1997). These tools have also been included because they address many of the problems which have been identified throughout this text concerning the interaction which occurs currently between women who experience domestic violence and healthcare professionals.

Notes

[1] For example, shifts in concepts of subjectivity as found in the work of Foucault (1990, 1991) and the relationship between the scientific project and medicine (Zola, 1977; Szasz, 1961).

[2] This is not surprising considering how difficult it is to get domestic violence on the medical and health course curriculums in order to ensure that healthcare professionals (as other professionals) are trained in domestic violence awareness as a matter of course.

[3] Stanko et al (1998) did identify 26 case histories/vignettes as identified within public sector records. This suggests that standardised patients might be acceptable if a range of diversities were included.

[4] Within Britain a number of inter-agency initiatives have focused on domestic violence and health and have engaged healthcare professionals in general domestic violence training courses: for example, Hammersmith and Fulham, Leeds Inter-Agency group, and Derby Domestic Violence Action Group.

[5] This medical power and control wheel is reproduced from training material copyrighted by Cosgrove (1992). It is similar in design and intent to the 'power and control wheel' developed by Pence and Paymar (1986).

Summary to Part Three

This section has examined the issues of intra- and inter-agency collaboration and training in order to identify the professional ideologies which influence medical practice. It has also examined the interactions which occur between healthcare professionals in order to further highlight the existence of power within the medical hierarchy. In relation to training, Chapter Thirteen suggested that poor inter-agency collaboration is partly due to the way in which medical training is based on a biomedical rather than an holistic community-based model of learning. On a more positive note, it has also been suggested that moves towards more community-based training will facilitate better inter-agency working, as well as ensuring that issues such as domestic violence are incorporated in problem-based learning approaches. All three of these issues are inter-related and need to be incorporated into training in order to maximise the impact of any initiatives which attempt to address healthcare professionals' current lack of knowledge about domestic violence.

Box 11 identifies key issues relevant to healthcare professions engaging within an inter-agency context (see over).

Box 11: Key points concerning intra/inter-agency collaboration and training

Healthcare professionals should:

- Be aware of the roles of other health practitioners.

- Examine the potential which specific health providers already have to address domestic violence within their casework.

- Ensure that such professionals have the power and resources to act on their findings.

- Improve communication with secondary services by acting on information received.

- Consider their representation on multi-agency domestic violence forums.

- Look at the types of support networks which they utilise in order to alleviate professional frustration.

- Examine where they would access information about other services.

- Consider their use of other professional groups and whether direct access to certain services would improve relationships with others.

- Access post-qualifying domestic violence training.

- Consider the inter-agency collaboration skills of prospective additions to health teams.

- Encourage the use of community/problem-based learning in training exercises.

- Examine available domestic violence tools in order to identify those which would assist in clinical practice.

- Use and disseminate such tools as appropriate.

FOURTEEN

Conclusion

The following five key findings emerged throughout this research. These points relate to the summaries of recommendations and 'good practice' which are located at the end of each results section.

1. Women present to healthcare professionals for the validation of their experiences.

Due to a lack of uniformity in treatment options, not least as a result of a lack of information and knowledge about domestic violence, women do not feel that they have their experiences validated, and therefore are critical of the medical interactions which take place. Women who experience domestic violence want their experiences validated in the health interaction. If this does not occur within an holistic/person-led approach then they may resort to activities intended to locate them within a biomedical context. Health practitioners need to be aware, therefore, of how patients perceive their ability to appropriate the sick role and ensure that validation is forthcoming for patients who may subsequently alter their behaviour in order to achieve this appropriation.

2. There was a clear differentiation made between the identification, documentation and treatment of physical and non-physical injuries.

While healthcare professionals are competent at identifying physical injuries, whether they act on this identification or not, and are also capable of recognising psychosomatic manifestations of domestic violence-related injuries, they were uncomfortable and reluctant to acknowledge the significance of self-harm and para-suicidal activity in relation to domestic violence. This resulted, in the most extreme cases, in women self-medicating in order to avoid health interactions where their search for validation went unheard.

3. Healthcare professionals use cultural myths and stereotypes about women who experience domestic violence which perpetuate their professional frustrations relating to the treatment of domestic violence-related injuries.

The frustrations which healthcare professionals experienced were compounded by the explanations they used to account for domestic violence, as well as by the expectations they had about women being in a position to prevent future injuries. This finding clearly challenges the effectiveness of social awareness campaigns (such as Zero Tolerance) and the media generally at targeting professional practice through social responsibilities.

4. The existence of a medical hierarchy undermines the potential of non-medical health professionals to interact positively with women who have domestic violence-related injuries.

This is unfortunate, as it is predominantly non-medical health personnel who are represented in inter-agency initiatives (where health representation does actually exist). Health visitors in particular are ideally placed to address the issue of domestic violence, but must be fully integrated within medical teams in order to maximise their clinical potential. The lack of inter-agency collaboration by healthcare professionals negates an understanding of the wider help-seeking processes which women who experience domestic violence engage in. It increases the frustrations which healthcare professionals feel, by isolating them from existing sources of information, and undermines the contribution they may be able to make by silencing the clinical practice and experiences of various health professions.

5. Domestic violence, in and of itself, has not undergone medicalisation and is unlikely to.

This is due to the way in which many of the symptoms of domestic violence have already undergone medicalisation in relation to the position of women in medical discourse. Domestic violence is, however, a serious public health issue, and requires a medical response which offers health practitioners an opportunity to move towards more holistic community-based health services which are more compatible with the treatment of social problems, whether they have undergone a process of medicalisation or not.

It is important that medical practitioners consider their professional practice in light of a number of contexts, in order to improve the services currently offered to women who present to healthcare professionals with violence-related injuries. First, this text has shown that women's help seeking from health practitioners cannot be isolated from wider help-seeking activities. Health professionals therefore need an understanding of multi-agency fora. This understanding would also give practitioners an opportunity to gain access to localised information about service provision, as well as offering support to deal with the frustrations that they face.

Second, the participating women's help seeking takes place in the context of domestic violence itself. This has important ramifications for the subjectivity of the presenting patient. This may manifest itself in the individual's behaviour and/or attitude generally. It may also limit her choices in relation to treatment options. Practitioners need to be aware, therefore, of the impact of domestic violence. This knowledge, as demonstrated in this book, is available from the testimonies of those who have experienced domestic violence. It is important that these voices remain central to any health initiatives intended to improve practice. Only through ongoing communication between patients and health providers will appropriate responses be developed and implemented. As highlighted in the key findings above, women will avoid professional contact if such experience compounds their experience of domestic violence itself. This is both frustrating for healthcare professionals and dangerous to the health and well-being of women who experience domestic violence. Acknowledging and understanding what domestic violence is, in relation to abuses of power and control, should be central to any health interaction which takes place.

Finally, domestic violence and the health interaction both take place within a wider social context. This has been demonstrated in relation to the ways in which cultural myths and stereotypes impact on clinical practice, and in relation to women's attempts to appropriate the sick role. As more professionals begin to address domestic violence within their caseloads and dialogue continues through multi-agency forums, the landscape of domestic violence, and our social understanding of it, is shifting. It is important for health professionals and the medical discourse as a whole that they are instrumental, both as professionals and as social citizens, within these dialogues.

Bibliography

Abbott, J., Johnson, R., Koziol, J., McLain, S. and Lowenstein (1995) 'Domestic violence against women: incidence and prevalence in an emergency department population', *Journal of the American Medical Association*, vol 273, no 22, pp 1763-7.

Abbott, P. and Williamson, E. (1999) 'Women, health and domestic violence', *Journal of Gender Studies*, vol 8, no 1, p 83-102.

Aldarondo, E. and Straus, M.A. (1994) 'Screening for physical violence in couple therapy: methodological, practical, and ethical considerations', *Family Process*, vol 33, pp 425-39.

AMA (American Medical Association) (1992) 'AMA diagnostic and treatment guidelines on domestic violence', *Archive of Family Medicine*, vol 1, 1 September, pp 39-47.

Amnesty International (1994) *Ethical codes and declarations relevant to the health professions: An Amnesty International compilation of selected ethical texts*, Amnesty International, 1 Easton Street, London, WC1X 8DJ, UK.

Astin, M., Lawrence, K. and Foy, D. (1993) 'Post traumatic stress disorder among battered women: risk and resiliency factors', *Violence and Victims*, vol 8, pp 17-28.

BAAMA (British Association of Accident and Emergency Medicine) (1994) *Domestic violence: Recognition and management in accident and emergency*, London: Royal College of Surgeons.

Bancroft, J., Skrimshire, A., Casson, J., Harvard-Watts, O. and Reynolds, F. (1977) 'People who deliberately poison or injure themselves: their problems and contacts with helping agencies', *Psychological Medicine*, vol 7, pp 289-303.

Bart, P.B. and Moran, E.G. (1993) *Violence against women: The bloody footprints*, London: Sage Publications.

Bates, L., Redman, S., Brown, W. and Hancock, L. (1995) 'Domestic violence experienced by women attending an accident and emergency department', *Australian Journal of Public Health*, vol 19, no 3, pp 293-9.

Becker, H.S. and McCall, M. (1990) *Symbolic interaction and cultural studies*, London: Chicago University Press.

Berg, M. (1996) 'Practices of reading and writing: the constitutive role of the patient record in medical work', *Sociology of Health and Illness*, vol 18, no 4, pp 499-524.

Bergman, B. and Brismar, B. (1991) 'Suicide attempts by battered wives', *Acta Psychiatr Scand*, vol 83, pp 380-4.

Billingham, K. and Hall, D. (1998) 'Turbulent future for school nursing and health visiting: change the bathwater – but hang on to the baby', *British Medical Journal*, vol 316, pp 406-7.

BMA (British Medical Association) (1998) *Domestic violence: A health care issue?*, London: BMA.

Bograd, M. (1982) 'Battered women, cultural myth and clinical interventions: a feminist analysis', *Women and Therapy*, vol 1, no 3, pp 69-77.

Bridgeman, C. and Hobbs, L. (1997) *Preventing repeat victimisation: The police officers guide*, Police Research Series, Policing and Reducing Crime Unit, London: Home Office.

B Team, The (1994) *Working with men who batter their partners (An introductory text)*, published by Working with men/The B Team, 320 Commercial Way, London SE15 1QN.

Budd, S. and Sharma, U. (eds) (1994) *The healing bond: The patient–practitioner relationship and therapeutic responsibility*, London: Routledge.

Butler, M.J. (1995) 'Domestic violence: a nursing imperative', *Journal of Holistic Nursing*, vol 13, no 1, pp 54-69.

Byrne, G. and Heyman, R. (1997) 'Understanding nurses' communication with patients in accident and emergency departments using a symbolic interactionist perspective', *Journal of Advanced Nursing*, vol 26, pp 93-100.

Campbell, J.C. (1992) 'Ways of teaching, learning and knowing about violence against women', *Nursing and Health Care*, vol 13, no 9, pp 464-70.

Candib, L.M.(1994) 'Self-in-relation theory: implications for women's health', in A.J. Dan (ed) *Reframing women's health: Multidisciplinary research and practice*, London: Sage.

Carmen, E., Rieker, P.P. and Mills, T. (1984) 'Victims of violence and psychiatric illness', *American Journal of Psychiatry*, vol 141, no 3, pp 378-83.

Cascardi, M., Langhinrichsen, J. and Vivian, D. (1992) 'Marital aggression: impact, injury and health correlates for husbands and wives', *American Medical Association*, vol 152, pp 1178-84.

Chez, N. (1994) 'Helping the victim of domestic violence', *American Journal of Nursing*, vol 94, no 7, pp 32-7.

Cloward, R.A. and Piven, F. (1979) 'Hidden protest: the channelling of female innovation and resistance', *Signs*, vol 4, no 4, pp 651-69.

Coleman, V.E. (1994) 'Lesbian battering: the relationship between personality and the perpetration of violence', *Violence and Victims*, vol 9, no 2, pp 139-52.

Cosgrove, A. (1992) 'Medical power and control wheel and advocacy wheel', available from the Domestic Violence Project Inc 6308, 8th Ave, Kenosha, WI 53143, USA.

Crawford, R. (1977) 'You are dangerous to your health: the ideology and politics of victim blaming', *International Journal of Health Services*, vol 4, no 4, pp 663-80.

Cross, L. (1993) 'Body and self in feminine development: implications for eating disorders and delicate self-mutilation', *Bull Menninger Clinic*, vol 57, pp 41-68.

Dan, A.J. (1994) *Reframing women's health: Multidisciplinary research and practice*, London: Sage Publications.

Davidson, L., King, V., Garcia, J. and Marchant, S. (2000) *Reducing domestic violence ... What works? Health services*, Policing and Reducing Crime Unit briefing notes, London: Home Office.

Davis, A.G. (1979) 'An unequivocal change in policy: prevention health and medical sociology', *Social Science and Medicine*, vol 13a, pp 129-37.

Delahunta, E.A. (1995) 'Hidden trauma: the mostly missed diagnosis of domestic violence', *American Journal of Emergency Medicine*, vol 13, no 1, pp 74-6.

Denham, S. (1995) 'Confronting the monster of family violence', *Nursing Forum*, vol 30, no 3, pp 12-19.

Derbyshire Constabulary 'D' Division (1997) Statistics obtained from the Police Domestic Violence Unit, Derby.

Desjarlais, R. and Kleinman, A. (1997) 'Violence and well-being', *Social Science and Medicine*, vol 45, no 8, pp 1143-5.

Dobash, R.E. and Dobash, R.P. (1979) 'If you prick me do I not bleed?', *Community Care*, 3 May, pp 26-8.

Dobash, R.E. and Dobash, R.P. (1992) *Women, violence and social change*, London: Routledge.

DoH (Department of Health) (2000) *Domestic violence: A resource manual for health care professionals*, London: DoH.

Domestic Violence Forum: Hammersmith and Fulham (1998) *Domestic violence services directory*, Funded by West London Health Promotion Agency, London: Hammerprint.

Donahue, J.M. and McGuire, M.B. (1995) 'The political economy of responsibility in health and illness', *Social Science and Medicine*, vol 40, no 1, pp 47-53.

Doner, K. (1994) 'Why violence is a health-care priority', *Social Policy*, vol 24, no 3, pp 58-62.

Douglas, M. (1994) 'The construction of the physician: a cultural approach to medical fashions', in S. Budd and U. Sharma (eds) *The healing bond: The patient–practitioner relationship and therapeutic responsibility*, London: Routledge.

Drake, V.K. (1982) 'Battered women: a health care problem in disguise', *Image* , vol 14, pp 45-6.

Dutton, D. and Painter, S.L. (1981) 'Traumatic bonding: the development of emotional attachments in battered women and other relationships of intermittent abuse', *Victimology: An International Journal*, vol 6, nos 1-4, pp 139-55.

Dworkin, A. (1983) *Right wing women*, London: Women's Press.

Dym, H. (1995) 'The abused patient', *Dental Clinics of North America*, vol 39, no 3, pp 621-35.

Easteal, P.W. (1994) *Voices of the survivors: Powerful and moving stories from survivors of sexual assault*, North Melbourne: Spinifex.

Easteal, P.W. and Easteal, S. (1992) 'Attitudes and practices of doctors toward spouse assault victims: an Australian study', *Violence and Victims*, vol 7, no 3.

Edleson, J.L. and Tolman, R.M. (1992) *Intervention for men who batter: An ecological approach*, London: Sage Publications.

Edwards, S. (1986) *The Police response to domestic violence in London*, London: Central London Polytechnic.

Eisikovits, Z.C. and Edleson, J.L. (1989) 'Intervening with men who batter: a critical review of the literature', *Social Service Review*, September, vol 37, pp 384-414.

Favazza, A.R. (1996) *Bodies under siege: Self-mutilation and body modification in culture and psychiatry*, London: John Hopkins University Press.

Ferraro, K.J. and Johnson, J.M. (1983) 'How women experience battering: the process of victimisation', *Social Problems*, vol 30, no 3, pp 325-39.

Finerman, R. and Bennett, L.A. (1995) 'Guilt, blame and shame: responsibility in health and sickness', *Social Science and Medicine*, vol 40, no 1, pp 1-3.

Finkler, K. (1997) 'Gender, domestic violence and sickness in Mexico', *Social Science and Medicine*, vol 45, no 8, pp 1147-60.

Fischbach, R.L. and Herbert, B. (1997) 'Domestic violence and mental health: correlates and conundrums within and across cultures', *Social Science and Medicine*, vol 45, no 8, pp 1161-76.

Fishwick, N. (1995) 'Nursing care of domestic violence victims in acute and critical care settings', *AACN Clinical Issues*, vol 6, no 1, pp 63-9.

Flexner, A. (1912) *Medical education in Europe*, New York, NY: Carnegie Foundation.

Foucault, M. (1990) *History of sexuality. Volume I: An introduction*, London: Penguin.

Foucault, M. (1991) *The birth of the clinic*, London: Routledge.

Freidson, E. (1970) *Profession of medicine: A study of applied knowledge*, London: Harper and Row.

Friend, J., Mezey, G. and Bewley, S. (1998) *Violence against women*, London: Royal College of Obstetrics and Gynaecology.

Gallagher, E.B. and Ferrante, J. (1987) 'Medicalization and social justice', *Social Justice Research*, vol 1, no 3, pp 377-92.

Gayford, J.J. (1975a) 'Battered wives', *Medicine, Science and Law*, vol 15, no 4, p 237.

Gayford, J.J. (1975b) 'Wife battering: a preliminary survey of 100 cases', *British Medical Journal*, vol 1, pp 194-7.

Glass, D.D. (1995) *All my fault*, London: Virago.

GMC (General Medical Council) (1993) *Tomorrow's doctors: Recommendations on undergraduate medical education*, London: GMC.

Goffman, E. (1968) *Stigma: Notes on the management of spoiled identity*, Harmondsworth: Penguin.

Goldberg, W.G. and Tomlanovich, M.C. (1984) 'Domestic violence victims in the emergency department', *Journal of the American Medical Association*, vol 251, pp 3259-64.

Gondolf, E.W. (1998) *Assessing woman battering in mental health services*, London: Sage Publications.

Goodwin, J. (1985) 'Family violence: principles of intervention and prevention', *Hospital and Community Psychiatry*, vol 36, pp 1074-9.

Grant, A., Niyonsenga, T. and Bernier, R. (1994) 'The role of medical informatics in health promotion and disease prevention', *Generations*, Spring, vol 18, no 1, pp 74-7.

Griffiths, S. (1998) 'From health to health care', *British Medical Journal*, vol 316, pp 296-301.

Hadley, S.M. (1992) 'Working with battered women in the emergency department: a model program', *Journal of Emergency Nursing*, vol 18, no 1, pp 18-23.

Hague, G. and Malos, E. (1993) *Domestic violence: Action for change*, Cheltenham: New Clarion Press.

Hague, G., Malos, E. and Dear, W. (1996) *Multi-agency work and domestic violence: A national study of inter-agency initiatives*, Bristol: The Policy Press.

Hamlin, E.R., Elwood, R., Donneworth, D. and Georgoulakis, J.M. (1991) 'A survey of army medical department personnel beliefs about domestic violence', *Military Medicine*, vol 156, no 9, pp 474-9.

Hanmer, J. and Maynard, M. (1987) *Women, violence and social control*, Explorations in Sociology 23, London: British Sociological Association/Macmillan.

Hanmer, J., Griffiths, S. and Jerwood, D. (1999) *Arresting evidence: Domestic violence and repeat victimisation*, Police Research Series Paper 104, Policing and Reducing Crime Unit, London: Home Office.

Harwin, N. (1997) Discussion extracts, J. Friend, G. Mezey and S. Bewley (1998) *Violence against women*, London: Royal College of Obstetrics and Gynaecology.

Hastings, J.E. and Hamberger, L.K. (1988) 'Personality characteristics of spouse abusers: a controlled comparison', *Violence and Victims*, vol 3, no 1, pp 31-48.

Heath, I. (1992) *Domestic violence: The general practitioner role*, London: Sabrecrown.

Heise, L.L. (1994) 'Gender-based abuse: the global epidemic', in A.J. Dan (ed) *Reframing women's health*, London: Sage Publications.

Heise, L.L., Raikes, A., Watts, C.H. and Zwi, A.B. (1994) 'Violence against women: a neglected public health issue in less developed countries', *Social Science and Medicine*, vol 39, no 9, pp 1165-79.

Hendricks-Matthews, M.K. (1993) 'Survivors of abuse: health care issues', *Family violence and abusive relationships*, vol 20, no 2, pp 391-405.

Herman, J.L. (1992a) *Trauma and recovery*, New York, NY: Basic Books.

Herman, J.L. (1992b) 'Complex PTSD: a syndrome in survivors of prolonged and repeated trauma', *Journal of Traumatic Stress*, vol 5, no 3, pp 377-91.

Hester, M. and Radford, L. (1996) *Domestic violence and child contact arrangements in England and Denmark*, Bristol: The Policy Press.

Hester, M., Pearson, C. and Radford, L. (1996) *Domestic violence: A national survey of court welfare and voluntary sector mediation practice*, Bristol: The Policy Press.

Hester, M., Pearson, C. and Harwin, L. (1998) *Making an impact: Children and domestic violence: A reader*, Bristol: University of Bristol/ Barnardo's/ NSPCC, Copies available from NSPCC training, Leicester.

Hite, S. (1977) *The Hite report: A nationwide study of female sexuality*, London: Summit.

Hoeg-Apel, C.M. (1994) 'Protocol for domestic violence intervention', *Nursing Management*, vol 25, no 9, pp 81-2.

Home Office (1989) *Domestic violence*, Home Office Research Study 107, London: HMSO.

Home Office (1995) *Inter-agency circular: Inter-agency co-ordination to tackle domestic violence*, London: Home Office.

House, R. (1996) 'General practice counselling: a plea for ideological engagement', *Counselling*, February.

House, R. (1997) 'The dynamics of professionalism: a personal view of counselling research', *Counselling*, August.

Housekamp, B.M. and Foy, D.W. (1991) 'The assessment of posttraumatic stress disorder in battered women', *Journal of Interpersonal Violence*, vol 6, pp 367-75.

Hudson-Allez, G. (1997) *Time-limited therapy in a general practice setting: How to help within six sessions*, London: Sage Publications.

Hughes, D. (1988) 'When nurse knows best: some aspects of nurse/ doctor interaction in a casualty department', *Sociology of Health and Illness*, vol 10, no 1, pp 1-22.

Illich, I. (1976) *Limits to medicine: Medical nemesis: The expropriation of health*, Harmondsworth: Penguin.

Illich, I., Zola, I.K., McKnight, J., Caplan, J. and Shaiken, H. (eds) (1977) *Disabling professions*, London: Marion Boyars.

Jeffery, R. (1979) 'Normal rubbish: deviant patients in casualty departments', *Sociology of Health and Illness*, vol 1, no 1, pp 90-107.

Johnson, K.K. (1979) 'Durkheim revisited: "Why do women kill themselves?"', *Suicide and Life-Threatening Behaviour*, vol 9, no 3, pp 145-53.

Johnson, L.A. (1995) 'Spurious assumptions about emergency department domestic violence victim caseloads', *Annals of Emergency Medicine*, vol 25, no 4, pp 561-2.

Kelly, D. (1997) 'Patients as partners in medical education', in C. Whitehouse, M. Roland and P. Campion (eds) *Teaching medicine in the community: A guide for undergraduate education*, Oxford General Practice Series no 38, Oxford.

Kelly, L., Bindel, J., Burton, S., Butterworth, D., Coch, K. and Regan, L. (1999) *Domestic violence matters: An evaluation of a development project*, Home Office Research Study 193, London: Home Office.

Kelly, L. (2000) *Reducing domestic violence ... what works? Outreach and advocacy approaches*, Policing and Reducing Crime Unit briefing notes, London: Home Office.

Kelner, M. and Wellman, B. (1997) 'Health care and consumer choice: medical and alternative therapies', *Social Science and Medicine*, vol 45, no 2, pp 203-12.

King, K.B., Parrinello, K.M. and Baggs, J.G. (1996) 'Collaboration and advanced practice nursing', in J.V. Hickey, R.M. Ouimette and S.L. Venegoni (eds) *Advanced practice nursing: Changing roles and clinical applications,* Philadelphia, PA: Lippincott-Raveri.

Kinkhorst, O.M., Alleman, A.W. and Hasman, A. (1996) 'From medical record to patient record through electronic data interchange (EDI)', *International Journal of Bio-Medical Computing*, vol 42, nos 1-2, pp 151-5.

Klingbeil, K.S. (1986) 'Interpersonal violence: a hospital based model from policy to program', *Response,* vol 9, no 3, pp 6-9.

Klingbeil, K.S. and Boyd, V.D. (1984) 'Emergency room intervention: detection, assessment and treatment', in A.R. Roberts (ed) *Battered women and their families: Intervention strategies and treatment programs,* New York, NY: Springer.

Kornblit, A.L. (1994) 'Domestic violence – an emerging health issue', *Social Science and Medicine*, vol 39, no 9, pp 1181-8.

Koss, M.P. (1994) 'The negative impact of crime victimization on women's health and medical use', in A.J. Dan (ed) *Reframing women's health: Multidisciplinary research and practice*, London: Sage Publications.

Kristeva, J. (1982) *Powers of horror: An essay on abjection*, Columbia: Columbia University Press.

Kurz, D. (1987) 'Emergency department responses to battered women: resistance to medicalization', *Social Problems*, vol 34, pp 69-81.

Kurz, D. and Stark, E. (1988) 'Not so benign neglect: the medical response to battering', in K.Yllo and M. Bograd (eds) *Feminist perspectives on wife abuse*, London: Sage Publications.

Langford, D.R. (1990) 'Consotia: a strategy for improving the provision of health care to domestic violence survivors', *Response*, vol 13, no 1, pp 17-19.

Lazzaro, M.V. and McFarlane, J. (1991) 'Establishing a screening program for abused women', *Journal of Nursing Administration*, vol 21, no 10, pp 24-9.

Lennox, A. and Petersen, S. (1998) 'Development and evaluation of a community based, multi agency course for medical students: descriptive study', *British Medical Journal*, vol 316, pp 596-9.

Letellier, P. (1994) 'Gay and bisexual male domestic violence victimization: challenges to feminist theory and responses to violence', *Violence and Victims*, vol 9, no 2, pp 95-106.

Llewellyn, T., Roden, R. and O'Neill, V. (1995) 'Support for victims of assaults and domestic violence: are accident and emergency departments doing enough?', *Journal of Accident and Emergency Medicine*, vol 12, pp 32-3.

Lloyd, A. (1995) *Doubly deviant, doubly damned: Society's treatment of violent women*, London: Penguin.

Lorentlen, S. and Løkke, G. (1997) *Promoting equality: A common issue for men and women, Report on sub-theme 2A: Men's violence against women: The need to take responsibility*, Strasbourg: Council of Europe.

Loseke, D.R. and Cahill, S.E. (1984) 'The social construction of deviance: experts on battered women', *Social Problems*, vol 31, no 3, pp 296-310.

Lowenberg, J.S. and Davis, F. (1994) 'Beyond medicalisation – demedicalisation: the case of holistic health', *Sociology of Health and Illness*, vol 16, no 5.

Lupton, D. (1997) 'Doctors on the medical profession', *Sociology of Health and Illness*, vol 19, no 4, pp 480-97.

Lyons, A.S. and Petrucelli, R.J. (1987) *Medicine: An illustrated history*, New York, NY: Abrahms.

Mama, A. (1996) *The hidden struggle: Statutory and voluntary sector responses to violence against black women*, London: Whiting and Birch.

Maris, R.W. (1971) 'Deviance as therapy: the paradox of the self-destructive female', *Journal of Health and Social Behaviour*, June, vol 12, pp 113-24.

Marshall, M.N. (1998) 'Qualitative study of educational interaction between general practitioners and specialists', *British Medical Journal*, vol 316, pp 442-5.

McAfee, R.E. (1994) 'We need you in the fight against family violence', *Journal of Medical Association of Georgia*, vol 83, no 7, pp 400-2.

McDowell, J.D. (1994) 'Domestic violence: recognizing signs of abuse in patients', *Dental Teamwork*, vol 7, no 3, pp 23-5.

McGibbon, A., Cooper, L. and Kelly, L. (1989) *What support? Hammersmith and Fulham Council community police committee domestic violence project*, London: Hammersmith and Fulham Community Safety Unit.

McIlwaine, G. (1989) 'Women victims of domestic violence: treatment should extend beyond the obvious physical trauma', *British Medical Journal*, vol 299, 21 October, pp 995-6.

McWilliams, M. and McKiernan, G. (1993) *Bringing it out into the open: Domestic violence in Northern Ireland*, Belfast: HMSO.

Mercy, J.A. and Saltzman, L.E. (1989) 'Fatal violence among spouses in the United States, 1976-85', *American Journal of Public Health*, vol 79, no 5, pp 595-9.

Miles, A. (1988) *Women and mental illness*, Brighton: Wheatsheaf.

Miles, A. (1991) *Women, health and medicine*, Bristol: Open University Press.

Mill, J.S. (1929) *The subjection of women*, London: J.M. Dent and Sons.

Mullender, A. (2000a) *Reducing domestic violence ... what works? Meeting the needs of children*, Policing and Reducing Crime Unit briefing notes, London: Home Office.

Mullender, A. (2000b) *Reducing domestic violence ... what works? Perpetrator programmes*, Policing and Reducing Crime Unit briefing notes, London: Home Office.

Mullender, A., Kelly, L., Hague, G., Malos, E. and Imam, U. (2000) *Children's needs, coping strategies and understanding of woman abuse*, ESRC Report, Warwick: Department of Social Policy and Social Work, University of Warwick.

NIMH (National Institute of Mental Health) (1981) 'Characteristics of admission to selected mental health facilities', National Institute of Mental Health series CN, no 2, Washington, DC: US Printing Office.

Norton, L.B., Peipert, J.F., Zierler, S., Lima, B. and Hume, L. (1995) 'Battering in pregnancy: an assessment of two screening methods', *Obstetrics and Gynecology*, vol 85, no 3, pp 321-5.

Oakley, A. (1981) *From here to maternity – Becoming a mother*, Harmondsworth: Penguin.

Oakley, A. (1993) *Essays on women, medicine and health*, Edinburgh: Edinburgh University Press.

Oakley, A. (1984) *The captured womb: A history of the medical care of pregnant women*, Oxford: Basil Blackwell.

Olavarrieta, C. and Soleto, J. (1996) 'Domestic violence in Mexico', *Journal of the American Medical Association*, vol 275, no 24, pp 1937-41.

Osler, W. (1951) 'The student life', in *A way of life and selected writings of Sir William Osler*, New York, NY: Dover.

Pahl, J. (ed) (1985) *Private violence and public policy: The needs of battered women and the response of the public service*, London: Routledge and Kegan Paul.

Pahl, J. (1995) 'Health professionals and violence against women', in P. Kingston and B. Penhale (eds) *Family violence and the caring professions*, London: Macmillan.

Parsons, T. (1951) *The social system*, London: Routledge and Kegan Paul.

Parsons, L.H., Zaccaro, D., Wells, B., Stovall, T.G., Pearse, W.H. and Horger, E.O. (1995) 'Methods of and attitudes toward screening obstetrics and gynaecology patients for domestic violence', *American Journal of Obstetrics and Gynecology*, vol 173, no 2, pp 381-7.

Pence, E. and Paymar, M. (1986) *Power and control: Tactics of men who batter*, Duluth, MN: Domestic Abuse Intervention Project.

Peters, S., Stanley, I., Rose, M. and Salmon, P. (1998) 'Patients with medically unexplained symptoms: sources of patients' authority and implications for demands on medical care', *Social Science and Medicine*, vol 46, no 4-5, pp 559-65.

Phillips, A. and Rakusen, J. (1989) *The new our bodies ourselves*, Boston, MA: Women's Health Book Collective.

Pizzey, E. (1974) *Scream quietly or the neighbours will hear*, Cambridge: Cambridge University Press.

Pizzey, E. and Shapiro, R.J. (1982) *Prone to violence*, London: Hamlyn.

Plotnikoff, J. and Woolfson, R. (1998) *Policing domestic violence: Effective organisational structures*, Policing and Reducing Crime, Police Research Series Paper 100, London: Home Office.

Post, R.D., Willeit, A.B., Franks, R.D., House, R.M., Back, S.M. and Weissberg, M.P. (1980) 'A preliminary report on the prevalence of domestic violence among psychiatric inpatients', *American Journal of Psychiatry*, vol 137, no 8, pp 974-5.

Ptacek, J. (1988) 'Why do men batter their wives?', in K. Yllo and M. Bograd (eds) *Feminist perspectives on wife abuse*, London: Sage Publications.

Radford, J. (1987) 'Policing male violence – policing women', in J. Hanmer and M. Maynard (eds) *Women, violence and social control*, Explorations in Sociology 23, London: British Sociological Association/ Macmillan.

Radford, J. (1992) 'Womanslaughter: a license to kill? The killing of Jane Asher', in J. Radford and D.E.H. Russell (eds) *Femicide: The politics of woman killing*, Buckingham: Open University Press.

Radford, J. and Russell, D.E.H. (1992) *Femicide: The politics of woman killing*, Buckingham: Open University Press.

Randall, T. (1990a) 'Domestic violence intervention calls for more than treating injuries', *Journal of the American Medical Association*, vol 264, no 8, pp 939-40.

Randall, T. (1990b) 'Domestic violence begets other problems of which physicians must be aware to be effective', *Journal of the American Medical Association*, vol 264, no 8, pp 943-4.

Richardson, J. and Feder, G. (1996) 'Domestic violence: a hidden problem for general practice', *British Journal of General Practice*, vol 46, pp 239-42.

Riessman, C.K. (1983) 'Women and medicalization: a new perspective', *Social Policy*, vol 14, no 1, pp 3-18.

Roy, M. (1977) 'A current survey of 150 cases', in M. Roy (ed) *Battered women: A psychosociological study of domestic violence*, New York, NY: Van Nostrand Reinhold.

Salmon, P., Sharma, N., Valori, R. and Bellenger, N. (1994) 'Patients' intentions in primary care: relationship to physical and psychological symptoms, and their perception by general practitioners', *Social Science and Medicine*, vol 38, no 4, pp 585-92.

Sanders, S.J. and Sonkin, D.J. (1995) 'Reporting obligations under the Vulnerable Adults Act', *Minnesota Medicine*, vol 78, no 9, pp 43-6.

Saunders, D.G. (1994) 'Post traumatic stress symptom profiles of battered women: a comparison of survivors in two settings', *Violence and Victims*, vol 9, no 1, pp 31-44.

Schneider, J.W. and Conrad, P. (1980) 'The medical control of deviance: contests and consequences', *Research in the Sociology of Health Care*, vol 1, pp 1-53.

Schoonmaker, J. and Shull, T. (1994) 'Domestic violence in the medical school curriculum', *Academic Medicine*, vol 69, no 5, p 412.

Schornstein, S.L. (1997) *Domestic violence and health care: What every professional needs to know*, London: Sage Publications.

Schur, E.M. (1984) *Labeling women deviant*, New York, NY: New York University, Random House.

Sharma, U. (1994) 'The equation of responsibility: complementary practitioners and their patients', in S. Budd and U. Sharma (eds) *The healing bond: The patient–practitioner relationship and therapeutic responsibility*, London: Routledge.

Sheridan, D.J. (1993) 'The role of the battered woman specialist', *Journal of Psychosocial Nursing*, vol 31, no 11, pp 31-7 and 46-7.

Sonkin, D.J. (1986) 'Clairvoyance vs common sense: therapists' duty to warn and protect', *Violence and Victims*, vol 1, no 1, pp 7-22.

Southon, G. and Braithwaite, J. (1998) 'The end of professionalism?', *Social Science and Medicine*, vol 46, no 1, pp 23-8.

Stanko, E.A. (1987) 'Typical violence, normal precaution: men, women and interpersonal violence in England, Wales, Scotland and the USA', in J. Hanmer and M. Maynard (eds) *Women, violence and social control*, Explorations in Sociology 23, London: British Sociological Association/ Macmillan.

Stanko, E.A. (1988) 'Fear of crime and the myth of the safe home: a feminist critique of criminology', in K. Yllo and M. Bograd (eds) *Feminist perspectives on wife abuse*, London: Sage Publications.

Stanko, E.A., Crisp, D., Hale, C. and Lucraft, H. (1998) *Counting the costs: Estimating the impact of domestic violence in the London Borough of Hackney*, Swindon: Crime Concern.

Stark, E. (1982) 'Doctors in spite of themselves: the limits of radical health criticism', *International Journal of Health Services*, vol 12, no 3, pp 419-57.

Stark, E. and Flitcraft, A. (1982) 'Medical therapy as repression: the case of the battered woman', *Health and Medicine*, vol 1, no 3, pp 29-32.

Stark, E. and Flitcraft, A. (1995) Killing the beast within: women battering and female suicidality', *International Journal of Health Services*, vol 25, no 1, pp 43-64.

Stark, E. and Flitcraft, A. (1996) *Women at risk: Domestic violence and women's health*, London: Sage Publications.

Stein, L. (1967) 'The doctor – nurse game', *Archives of General Psychiatry*, vol 16, pp 699-703.

Stimson, G. (1976) 'General practitioners, "trouble" and types of patient', in M. Stacey (ed) *The sociology of the NHS*, Sociological Review Monographs no 22, Keele: University of Keele Press.

Straus, M.A. and Smith, C. (1993) 'Family patterns and primary prevention of family violence', *Trends in Health Care, Law and Ethics*, vol 8, no 2, pp 17-25.

Svensson, R. (1996) 'The interplay between doctors and nurses – a negotiated order perspective', *Sociology of Health and Illness*, vol 18, no 3, pp 379-98.

Szasz, T. (1961) *The myth of mental illness*, New York, NY: Harper.

Taylor, G. (1994) 'Family violence and the community pharmacist', *American Pharmacy*, vol 34, no 4, pp 41-4.

Tilden, V.P. and Shepherd, P. (1987) 'Increasing the rate of identification of battered women in an emergency department: use of a nursing protocol', *Research in Nursing and Health*, vol 10, pp 209-15.

Tuan, Yi-Fu (1984) *Dominance and affection: The making of pets*, Yale: Yale University Press.

Tuckett, D., Boulton, M., Olson, C. and Williams, A. (1985) *Meetings between experts*, London and New York: Tavistock.

Turner, B.S. (1995) (2nd Edition) *Medical power and social knowledge*, London: Sage Publications.

UN (United Nations) (1993a) *Strategies for confronting domestic violence: A resource manual*, New York, NY: Washington Free Press.

UN (1993b) *Declaration on the elimination of violence against women*, New York, NY: Washington Free Press.

Varvaro, F.F. and Lasko, D.L. (1993) 'Physical abuse as cause of injury in women: information for orthopaedic nurses', *Orthopaedic Nursing*, vol 12, no 1, pp 37-41.

Vaughan, D. (1994) *Uncoupling: How and why relationships come apart*, London: Methuen (Cedar).

Walker, L.E.A. (1979) *The battered woman*, New York, NY: Harper and Row.

Walker, L.E.A. (1989) 'Psychology and violence against women', *American Psychologist*, vol 44, no 4, pp 695-702.

Walker, L.E.A. (1991) 'Post traumatic stress disorder in women: diagnosis and treatment of battered woman syndrome', *Psychotherapy*, vol 28, no 1, pp 21-9.

Walker, M. (1988) 'Training the trainers: socialisation and change in general practice', *Sociology of Health and Illness*, vol 10, no 3, pp 283-302.

Wallman, S. and Baker, M. (1996) 'Which resources pay for treatment? A model for estimating the informal economy of health', *Social Science and Medicine*, vol 42, no 5, pp 671-9.

Ward, M. and Loenenthal, D. (1997) 'Differential client referral patterns in the GP setting', *Counselling*, May, pp 129-31.

Warshaw, C. (1992) 'Domestic violence: challenges to medical practice', *Journal of Women's Health*, vol 2, no 1, pp 73-80.

Warshaw, C. (1994) 'Domestic violence: challenges to medical practice', in A.J. Dan (ed) *Reframing women's health: Multidisciplinary research and practice*, London: Sage Publications.

Weale, A. (1998) 'Rationing health care: a logical solution to an inconsistent triad', *British Medical Journal*, vol 316, pp 410.

Webster, J., Sweett, S. and Stolz, T.A. (1994) 'Domestic violence in pregnancy: a prevalence study', *The Medical Journal of Australia*, vol 17, pt 161, no 8, pp 466-70.

Whitehouse, C., Roland, M. and Campion, P. (eds) (1997) *Teaching medicine in the community: A guide for undergraduate education*, Oxford General Practice Series no 38, Oxford.

WHO (World Health Organisation) (1997) *Violence against women: A priority health issue*, Geneva: WHO.

Williamson, E. (1999) *Domestic violence and the response of the medical profession*, Doctoral thesis, Derby: University of Derby.

Williamson, E. (2000) 'Caught in contradictions: conducting feminist action oriented research within an evaluated research programme', in J. Radford, M. Friedberg and L. Harne (eds) *Women, violence, and strategies for action: Feminist research, policy and action*, Milton Keynes: Open University Press.

Wilson, M. and Daly, M. (1992) 'Till death us do part', in J. Radford and D.E.H. Russell (eds) *Femicide: The politics of woman killing*, Buckingham: Open University Press.

Wolf, N. (1991) *The beauty myth*, London: Vintage.

Wolfe, D.A. and Korsch, B. (1994) 'Witnessing domestic violence during childhood and adolescence: Implication for pediatric practice', *Pediatrics*, vol 94, pt 4, no 2, pp 594-9.

Wollstonecraft, M. (1929) *A vindication of the rights of women*, London: J.M. Dent and Sons.

Worrel, J. and Reiner, T. (1992) *Feminist perspectives in therapy*, Chichester: Wiley.

Wyatt, J.C. (1998) 'Will improved clinical information help realise the new NHS?', *British Medical Journal*, vol 316, pp 296-301.

Yllo, K. and Bograd, M. (1988) *Feminist perspectives on wife abuse*, London: Sage Publications.

Zola, I.K. (1977) 'Healthism and disabling medicalization', in I. Illich, I.K. Zola, J. McKnight, J. Caplan and H. Shaiken (eds) *Disabling professions*, London: Marion Boyars.

Zuckerman, B., Augustyn, M., Groves, B. and Parker, S. (1995) 'Silent victims revisited: the special case of domestic violence', *Pediatrics*, vol 96, no 3, pp 511-3.

Appendix 1
Details of research participants

Table A1: Demographic and autobiographical details of stage one participants

Name and occupation	Age range and ethnicity	Type of interview	Children	History of abuse	Mental health services	A & E	General practice
Amy Health care manager	46 British	One untaped formal interview	Two grown-up children	Lived with abuser for 23 years; experienced physical, emotional, sexual and psychological abuse	Had attempted suicide three times	Numerous presentations at A & E, both for own and children's injuries*	Consistently presented with injuries; did not disclose for fear of further violence
Brenda Unemployed due to ill health	27 British	One untaped informal interview	No children	Current partner had completed male intervention programme; previous partner had been abusive	Had had contact with mental-health services for depression, anxiety, and para-suicidal behaviour	Taken to A and E after suicidal activity	Was struck off from general practice for suicidal behaviour
Carol Single mother	32 West Indian descent British	Two taped formal interviews; one untaped informal interview	Four boys; the eldest was 15 and no longer lived with Carol	Lived with abusive partner for 16 years, who was also the father of her children	Had attempted suicide four times, and had contact with mental health services as a result	Several times including for stab wound, strangulation and damage to eyes	Frequent visits including while pregnant
Debbie Professional within voluntary sector	27 Asian descent British	Two taped formal interviews and numerous discussions	No children	Lived with psychologically abusive partner; also witnessed and experienced domestic violence as a child	Had contact with mental health services as a child for suicidal activity, and as an adult for counselling	Was taken to A & E in relation to suicidal activity	Requested counselling and support on several occasions as a young woman; was struck off
Emma Administrator	24 Greek descent British	Two taped formal interviews	One baby	Has since married previously abusive boyfriend; did not experience physical violence	Contact with mental health services in relation to a single suicide attempt; also in relation to eating disorders	Once due to suicide attempt	Numerous occasions in relation to anxiety, depression, eating disorders
Frances Professional	32 British	One untaped informal interview and one taped interview	No biological children; one step-child	Experienced emotional and psychological abuse with previous partner	Contact with mental health services in relation to depression		Visited general practice in relation to depression
Georgina Unemployed	22 British	Two untaped informal interviews; issues arose concerning boundaries which negated further contact	No children	Experienced physically and psychologically abusive relationship over two years	Was taking antidepressants following a suicide attempt	In addition to suicide attempt, had gone concerning broken arm	Had visited general practice for general depression and anxiety

Table A1 cont.../: Demographic and autobiographical details of stage one participants

Name and occupation	Age range and ethnicity	Type of interview	Children	History of abuse	Mental health services	A & E	General practice
Helena Professional	49 Irish descent British	One taped formal interview and several discussions	Talked about one grown-up child; possibly other children whom Helena did not identify	Physically, sexually and emotionally abusive relationship	Had no contact with mental health services at the time; was now herself a counsellor	Attended A and E for numerous injuries	Visited general practice in relation to physical injuries
Iris Professional	42 British	One taped formal interview	One grown-up child who had remained with abusive partner	Was physically and psychologically abused shortly after getting married	Had contact with mental health services for general depression and anxiety at time of abusive relationship		Had visited general practice for a number of minor injuries as well as for broken ribs
Jemima Professional	23 British	Several short taped interviews	No children	Lived in an emotionally and psychologically abusive relationship for five years which ended with physical violence	Had attempted suicide	Was taken to A & E following suicide attempt; also for suspected fractured wrist	After physical violence went to general practice concerning suspected fractured wrist and was referred to A & E
Total:	Mean age = 32.4 years SD = 9.8 Range = 27	Seven taped interviews and three taped follow-up interviews were conducted; five untaped interviews	Five of the women had biological children, one had a step-child	All 10 women had experienced emotional and psychological abuse; eight women experienced at least one incident of physical abuse†, and four experienced sexual abuse	Nine out of 10 women had contact with mental health services; seven women had attempted suicide, three on multiple occasions	Seven of the women had visited A & E in relation to their para-suicidal activity, and five in relation to other physical injuries; 8 of the ten participating women had visited A & E in relation to their domestic violence-related injuries	All 10 women had contacted their GP, either for the treatment of physical injuries or in relation to anxiety and depression, or for referral to other services; two of the women had been 'struck off' from their GP surgeries

* This was pre-1989 Children's Act.

† Excluding Debbie's experience of abuse and domestic violence as a child.

Table A2: List of second stage participants

Name	Occupation	Gender	Type of practice	Number of patients	Number of practice nurses	Number of district nurses	Number of health visitors	Number of general practitioners	Number of counsellors/CPNs
Dr Aaron	GP	Male	Rural/town	6,000	2.5	0	2	3.5	0
Ms Babar	PN	Female	Single fundholding GP, inner city	2,500	1	0	0	1	0
Ms Cabourn*	HV	Female	Inner city	12,000	4	2	5 (base)	6	1
Ms Dabbs*	HV	Female	Inner city	12,000	4	2	5	6	1
Dr Eagland†	GP	Female	Rural/urban	10,000	2	0	2	6	1
Dr Fagan‡	GP	Male	Semi-rural	7,000	3	1	1		CPN
Dr Gabb	GP	Female	Urban/rural	9,000	3	3	2	4.5	0
Dr Habberley†	GP	Male	Rural/urban	10,000	2	0	2	6	1
Dr Iannelli	GP	Male	Inner city/urban	7,600	1.5	0	2	4	1
Dr Jabber	GP	Male	Suburban	6,000	1.5	1	1	3	0
Ms Kaberry	HV	Female	Mixed area	13,000	3	1	1	5	0
Ms Lacey	HV	Female	Urban	4,000	1	0	1	2.5	0
Dr McCabe	GP	Female	Town	3,000	1	0	1	1.5	0
Ms Naylor	PN	Female	Town	2,500	2	1	2	3	0
Ms O'Neill	PN	Female	Rural/urban	8,000	3	1	1	3.5	1
Dr Padden‡	GP	Male	Rural/urban	7,000	4	3	2	4	1
Dr Quadir	GP	Female	Mixed area	7,000	3	1	2	4	1
Ms Radcliffe	M	Female	Hospital	n/a	n/a	n/a	n/a	n/a	n/a
Ms Smith	C	Female	Inner city	n/a	n/a	n/a	n/a	n/a	n/a
Ms Taylor	C	Female	Inner city	n/a	n/a	n/a	n/a	n/a	n/a
Total:	GPs = 10 PN = 3 HV = 4 M = 1 C = 2	Male = 6 (GP) Female = 14	Inner city = 6 Town = 2 Hospital = 1 Mixed urban/rural = 9 Urban = 2	Mean = 7447 SD = 3292 Range = 2500-13,000	Mean = 2.4 Range = 1-4 SD = 1	Mean = 1 Range = 0-3 SD = 1	Mean = 1.94 Range = 0-5 SD = 1.298	Mean = 3.969 Range = 1-6 SD = 1.576	Mean = 0.529 Range = 0-1 SD = 0.514

Notes: * Same practice. † Same practice. ‡ Same practice.
GP = general practitioner; PN = practice nurse; HV = health visitor; M = midwife; C = counsellor.

Appendix 2
Useful information and contacts

Women's organisations

Women's Aid Federation of England
PO Box 391
Bristol BS99 7WS
Tel: 0117 944 4411 (office)
08457 023468 (helpline)
http://www.womensaid.org.uk

Welsh Women's Aid
38-48 Crwys Rd
Cardiff CF24 4NN
Tel: 029 2039 9874

*Black Association of Women
Step Out (BAWSO)*
109 St Mary St
Cardiff CF1 1DX
Tel: 01222 343154

Newham Asian Women's Project
661 Barking Rd
London E13 9EX

Southall Black Sisters
52 Norwood Rd
Southall
Middlesex UB2 4DW
Tel: 020 8571 9595

Refuge
2-8 Meltravers St
London WC2R 3EE
Tel: 020 7395 7700 (office)
0870 599 5443 (helpline)

Zero Tolerance Helpline
Tel: 0800 028 3398
0800 028 3397 (textphone)

Crime Reduction Unit

Copies of *Reducing domestic violence ... what works?*
briefing notes available from:
Policing and Reducing Crime Unit
Room 415, Clive House
Petty France
London SW1H 9HD.
http:/www.homeoffice.gov.uk/rds/index.htm

Home Office reports

Available from:
Information and Publications Group
Room 201, Home Office
50 Queen Anne's Gate
London SW1H 9AT
Tel: 020 7273 2084
http://www.homeoffice.gov.uk/domesticviolence

Department of Health

www.doh.gov.uk/domestic.htm

Copies of the DoH 'Domestic violence: a resource manual for health care professionals', available from:
DoH Publications
PO Box 777
London SE1 6XH
Fax: 01623 724524

General sites of interest

http://www.igc.apc.org/women/feminist.html
http://www.domesticviolencedata.org

ESRC violence programme

www.brunel.ac.uk/depts/law/dvds

World Health Organisation

http://www.who.int/